nth century saw                inning of

D1236666

**Guy Williams** was brought up in a predominantly medical family – his father, a country practitioner, naming him gratefully after the founder of the famous London hospital at which he had been a student.

He has lived and worked in London for over thirty years. During that time he has published a number of books on historical subjects, his books on the history of London's police being particularly valued. He broadcasts regularly on various aspects of London life and has recently published a guide to the joys of walking in London.

A selection of reviews of Guy Williams's **The age of agony: the art of healing, c 1700–1800**

'For years I have wished for a medical history of the 18th century, one which would be comprehensible to the general reader . . . Guy Williams's *The age of agony* is the nearest approach so far to what I have been hoping for.' Margaret Lane, *Daily Telegraph*

'A splendidly robust book, which rattles through a century of suffering and throws a great deal of light upon the splendour, the misery, the arrogance, and the humiliation of the 18th century.' John Delin, *Sunday Telegraph*

'The author has researched his book well and presents many interesting aspects of 18th century medicine laced with plenty of amusing anecdotes.' Neil O'Donoghue, *New Scientist*

'Entertaining and illuminating reading.' *The Lancet*

'Compulsive reading. Recommend it to your patients. They will complain no more.' John Illman, *General Practitioner*

'Refreshing and compassionate . . . an excellent book which can be recommended to the average reader.' *British Book News*

Guy Williams

# The Age of Miracles

## Medicine and Surgery
## in the Nineteenth Century

Constable
London

This b
the mc
and my

Guy Williams

# The Age of Miracles

Medicine and Surgery
in the Nineteenth Century

Constable
London

First published in Great Britain 1981
by Constable and Company Ltd
10 Orange Street London WC2H 7EG
Copyright © 1981 by Guy Williams
ISBN 0 09 462360 0
Set in Monophoto Garamond 12pt by
Servis Filmsetting Ltd, Manchester
Printed in Great Britain by
Ebenezer Baylis and Son Ltd
The Trinity Press, Worcester

This book is dedicated to the two doctors who have meant the most to me – my father, Owen Elias Williams, of Mold, and my brother Huw Owen Williams, of Leominster and Kingsland

# Contents

# *Illustrations*

# Acknowledgements

In compiling the material contained in this book, I have drawn on a wide variety of sources. I have found these books particularly informative, and acknowledge my debt to their authors and publishers:

Stanley Chapman, *Jesse Boot of Boots the Chemists*, Hodder and Stoughton, London, 1974; Sigmund Freud, *Charcot, Collected Papers*, Hogarth Press, London, 1948; R.J. Godlee, *Lord Lister*, Oxford University Press, 1924; Douglas Guthrie, *A History of Medicine*, Thomas Nelson and Sons, London, 1945; Geoffrey Keynes (Ed.), *Blood Transfusion*, Simpkin Marshall Ltd, London, 1949; David Le Vay, *The Life of Hugh Owen Thomas*, E. & S. Livingstone, Edinburgh and London, 1956; Wyndham E.B. Lloyd, *A Hundred Years of Medicine*, Duckworth and Company, London 1968; G. Ruthven Mitchell, *Homoeopathy*, W.H. Allen, London, 1975; A.R.G. Owen, *Hysteria, Hypnosis and Healing: The Work of J-M. Charcot*, Dennis Dobson, London, 1971; A. Turner, *Joseph, Baron Lister*, The Centenary Volume, Edinburgh, 1927; E.S. Turner, *Taking the Cure*, Michael Joseph, London, 1967; Frederick Watson, *Hugh Owen Thomas*, Oxford University Press, 1934; and Cecil Woodham-Smith, *Florence Nightingale*, Constable and Company, London, 1950.

Other sources are acknowledged in the Notes at the end of this book. Mrs Knight obtained many old and rare books for me, and I am deeply grateful to her.

# *Preface*

This book recounts the story of the great advances that were made in the art of healing during the nineteenth century. It has not, of course, been possible to consider the years 1800–99 in isolation, because much of the work that led to the most significant discoveries was carried out in previous decades, and many of the benefits that have accrued from those discoveries were not fully appreciated until our present century was well on its way.

Many people have helped with the preparation of this book. I am especially grateful to Mr Benjamin Glazebrook, who encouraged me to write a sequel to *The Age of Agony*. My thanks are due, too, to several archivists and public relations officers who gave me most valuable assistance when I was carrying out my preliminary researches – I would mention in particular Miss Kerling of St Bartholomew's Hospital, Mr J.H.E. Orde of Guy's Hospital and Mr R.W. Sharpington of St Thomas's Hospital. The Librarian and staff of the Wellcome Institute of the History of Medicine have gone to much trouble on my behalf. So, too, have Mrs Knight and her assistants at the East Sheen branch of the Richmond Libraries.

The illustrations are reproduced by permission of the Wellcome Institute.

# I

# The Age of Miracles

*I wish no living thing to suffer pain . . .*

PERCY BYSSHE SHELLEY, 1792–1822

For people living before the end of the eighteenth century, irremediable pain was part of the human condition. It was liable to be suffered at a moment's notice, and the scientific knowledge to relieve it did not exist. By the end of the nineteenth century, pain had become less inevitable, and could be to some extent controlled. Good health could be regarded as a normal state of being, to be expected and enjoyed by the vast majority of civilized people. In medicine, the century was an Age of Miracles. Any book that describes such a century must, inevitably, be a happy one.

When the nineteenth century started, there were still many medical practitioners who had been brought up in a climate of ideas that had not altered much since the time of Hippocrates. Some still believed that a patient's health might be affected by internal 'humours', and that those humours could best be treated by such traditional methods as blistering, cauterising, purging, the administration of powerful emetics, and the drawing off of blood. As late as the year 1833, blood-letting was still so popular in Europe that in that year forty one and a half million leeches had to be imported into France alone.

But by the year 1800 the structure of the human body was almost fully understood, thanks to new methods of microscopy and of making injections. Even more important than this anatomical knowledge was the knowledge of physiological processes that was being rapidly acquired, most notably in Germany. What had been happening?

At a number of centres in various parts of Europe, dedicated teachers had been insisting that accurate scientific knowledge should replace guesswork and superstition. Turin had been famous for this in the seventeenth century. As Turin had faded in importance, Leyden had flourished. A surgeon attached to the army of King William III – John Monro – had visited Leyden, studied there, had returned to Edinburgh, and had been appointed Professor of Anatomy and Surgery to the Surgeons' Company in that city. He had specially educated his son Alexander (born 1697) so that the young man could succeed him in the Chair of Anatomy. In the process, Alexander Primus had been sent to study at Leyden under the greatest clinical teacher in Europe, Hermann Boerhaave. Alexander Primus had been succeeded at Edinburgh by his son Alexander Secundus (born 1733), and Alexander Secundus had been followed, in his turn, by his son Alexander Tertius (born 1773).[1] Under four successive generations of the Monro family, Edinburgh had become almost as important a centre of medical research as Leyden. In London, meanwhile, men such as Sir William Cheselden and Percivall Pott had been keeping in close touch with their Scottish contemporaries; and Scotland had provided London with the greatest phenomenon of all – Doctor John Hunter.

## 2

# John Hunter

*Our fellow-countryman is a model of a man, quite fresh*
*from Natur's mould! . . . Rough he may be, So air our*
*Barrs. Wild he may be, So air our Buffalers . . .*

CHARLES DICKENS, 1812—70
*Martin Chuzzlewit*

John Hunter was born on 13 February 1728 at Long
Calderwood in Lanarkshire. He was the youngest of ten
children of another John Hunter who, according to a
contemporary report, was 'a man of intelligence, integrity
and anxious temperament'. The boy's grandfather was
largely responsible for the finances of the City of Glasgow.

When he was a lad, John Hunter despised book work. He
evaded his lessons and spent as much time as he could in the
sports and games of the countryside. Then, when he was
about seventeen, he was sent to stay with one of his sisters in
Glasgow. This sister was married to a cabinet-maker whose
business was not thriving at the time. The plan was that John
should provide general assistance in exchange for being
taught the rudiments of craftsmanship. The scheme worked.
John soon acquired considerable manual skill.

As John laboured in Glasgow, he heard glowing reports
of the achievements of his elder brother William, who was
working in London. William, the seventh of the Hunter
children, had been intended by his father to enter the Scottish
Church. The idea of signing the required Articles of Faith did
not appeal to the earnest young man, however, and in this
predicament he had gone for advice to William Cullen, who
was practising in the district as a surgeon. Cullen had offered
to take William into his house and to make him a 'resident
pupil'.

There is no doubt that Cullen was an outstandingly good instructor.[1] He moved on soon after to Glasgow where, it was recorded, he urged his students to observe as carefully as they could the natural progress of all diseases. He taught them to attempt to discriminate between important symptoms and irrelevant ones. And he also taught them to discriminate between changes that were the result of man-administered remedies and changes that were the result of 'the curative operations of Nature'. William Hunter had worked under Cullen's personal surveillance for three years. During that time the young man had been much influenced by his mentor's respect for scientific discovery. For the rest of his life, William Hunter referred to Cullen as 'a man to whom I owe most and love most of all men in the world'.

After these three years the time had come, Cullen saw, for Hunter to gain wider experience. So he arranged for his young assistant to go first to Edinburgh, where Hunter spend a winter studying under the Professor Monro of the time and other distinguished instructors, after which he was to go to London.

In London, Hunter had been engaged as an assistant by James Douglas, a Scottish physician who had graduated at Rheims and who, after that, had earned himself a considerable reputation as an anatomist. This was a fortunate encounter for Hunter, for Douglas helped his young associate to enter St George's Hospital as a pupil and to get from other experts further instruction in anatomy.

By this time, William Hunter had become a tireless seeker after anatomical truth. The first important results of his labours had been contained in a paper he had contributed in 1743 to the Royal Society on 'The Structure and Diseases of Articulating Cartileges'. Three years after that, he had been invited to lecture regularly on anatomical subjects to the Association of Naval Surgeons at their rooms in Covent Garden. In the spring of 1748 he had set off on a European tour, during which he had visited Leyden and had met the great German Professor of Anatomy Bernard Siegfried

Albinus (born 1697) and Albinus had shown him the very successful method he had evolved of making injections.

Shortly after William Hunter returned from this European tour, his unlettered younger brother John decided to travel from Glasgow to London to join him. The young man made the long journey south on horseback. The plan was that John should be allowed to work in William's dissecting room, which was now becoming quite celebrated. Soon after John arrived in London, William asked him to carry out a dissection of the muscles of a human arm, and John did this so competently that his elder brother felt able to trust him with the general supervision of the second-year students.

For ten years after that, the Hunter brothers worked together more or less harmoniously. During this time, the Hunters made several discoveries that were to be of vital importance in the developing science of medicine. They tested the absorbing power of veins; they studied the nature of pus; they examined the nasal and olfactory nerves; they established the position of the testis in the unborn child; and they investigated thoroughly the manner in which blood circulates in the placenta. It seems likely that the younger and comparatively inarticulate John Hunter made most of these discoveries, and that the older, more sophisticated and more vocal William recorded them and brought them to public attention. The older brother did in fact often tell people that he could claim no credit for most of the great work done by John. Needing as much assistance as he could get with his clinical lectures, it is probable that William offered to take John into partnership with him in the course of this decade, but in the *European Magazine* of October 1782 it was stated, on John Hunter's authority, that the young brother had declined this honour, as he was self-conscious and loathed speaking in public.[2]

Towards the end of the decade, friction grew between the brothers, as William became increasingly interested in obstetrics and gradually withdrew from general surgery.

John's range of interests, meanwhile, steadily widened. At last, in 1760, John's lungs became inflamed and he felt thoroughly depressed and out of sorts. In an attempt to shake himself out of this decline, he decided to separate himself from his older brother and to make a career on his own. From this time on, the Hunters have to be thought of as separate cases.

William, left by John, continued to lecture, assisted by a brilliant young man named William Hewson. At the same time, he was steadily forming a collection of anatomical and pathological subjects. By 1765, his collection had grown to such an extent that he started to play with the idea of building a special museum 'for the improvement of anatomy, surgery and physic'. In a memorial he sent to George Grenville, First Lord of the Treasury and Chancellor of the Exchequer, William offered to spend £7000 of his own money on the construction of such a building if he were given the necessary plot of ground, and if a Professorship of Anatomy were endowed in perpetuity. The suggestion was turned down, but Lord Shelburne proposed that the cost should be met by public subscription. He would lay down a thousand guineas himself, he said. After lengthy consideration, William, who had recently been appointed Physician-Extraordinary to the Queen, decided to go ahead with the venture entirely at his own expense. He bought a plot of ground in Great Windmill Street and on this he started to build a house which would have dissecting rooms, a lecture theatre, and extensive galleries. It was to become London's most notable medical school.

Meanwhile, to make a complete break with his brother John Hunter had accepted, in 1760, an appointment as Staff Surgeon in an expedition that was to be led by Viscount Keppel. The enterprise was aimed principally at the French outpost of Belle-Île-en-Mer. The ships sailed in 1761, and Surgeon Hunter, as ever insatiably curious, spent much of his time studying the conditions under which blood coagulates. In the following year he was attached to the British Army in

Portugal, and there he was able to examine as many gunshot wounds as he wished as well as making an extensive study of various kinds of inflammation.

In 1763, John Hunter returned to London. Greatly invigorated by his adventures abroad, he began to practise as a surgeon in Golden Square. He started to give lectures on anatomy and operative surgery, probably in an attempt to outshine his brother William, but his uncultured delivery did not impress his pupils and the classes he attracted were small. This left him with plenty of mental energy for his own researches into human comparative anatomy and for some intensive investigations into a wide variety of other subjects. 'My mind is like a beehive', he is said to have observed. In order to have plenty of room in which to conduct his increasingly complex experiments, Hunter bought two acres of land at Earl's Court and built a roomy house on the ground. He had to enlarge this house soon afterwards, in a vain attempt to keep pace with his own burgeoning interests. The house contained well-equipped dissecting rooms, tanks for macerating, or softening by soaking, specimens that he intended to dissect, and numerous other facilities for scientific research; and in the garden there was a pond in which Hunter kept oysters since he wanted to experiment with the artificial formation of pearls. Round this pond, he planted an ever-increasing number of skulls.

Since his boyhood days in East Lothian, John Hunter had been fascinated by animals, and the cages with which the grounds of the house at Earl's Court were plentifully supplied were always well-tenanted. Many of the animals Hunter had in his menagerie were very rare. A considerable proportion of the fees he earned from his surgical practice went on buying these expensive specimens, and once, it is alleged, he even had to borrow five guineas from King George III's bookseller in order to purchase a dying tiger. On more than one occasion he bought some remarkable beast and allowed it to be publicly exhibited, but always, when he did this, he insisted that the cadaver should be sent back to

Earl's Court if and when the animal expired. There he would be waiting for it with his knife.

Of all the animals in his collection, John Hunter seemed to like best those which had plenty of spirit. He was particularly fond of a little bull that came to him as a present from the Queen; and he grew even more attached to it after it had knocked him down. On another occasion, two leopards that he owned managed to escape from their cages and started to fight. Quite unperturbed, and although he was unarmed, Hunter managed to overpower the beasts and get them safely back behind bars.

John Hunter was working at this time with the utmost dedication. Every hour he could snatch from his surgical practice, other than the very few hours he needed for sleep, was devoted to dissection or to experiments, or to reflection on those experiments' results. His stamina and his powers of concentration were probably unprecedented in the fields of medical research. One of his contemporaries described him as 'standing for hours, motionless as a statue, except that, with a pair of forceps in each hand, he was picking asunder the connecting fibres of some structure he was studying'. Sir James Paget (1814–99) was only one of many authoritative historians who have referred to John Hunter as 'the founder of scientific surgery'. Unusually, the work he was doing was properly appreciated at the time – among other honours he received was the Fellowship of the Royal Society in 1767, and he was appointed Surgeon to the King in 1776.

When William Hunter's grand new Palace of Anatomy in Great Windmill Street was complete, he moved out of the large house in Jermyn Street in which he had been living, and his brother John moved into it. Here, John was able to take house pupils, each of whom would be bound to him for a period of five years, paying a premium of five hundred guineas for the privilege. Among the first of John Hunter's 'apprentices' – for that is really what they were – was Edward Jenner, of Berkeley, in Gloucestershire, later to discover the value of vaccination in the fight against smallpox.

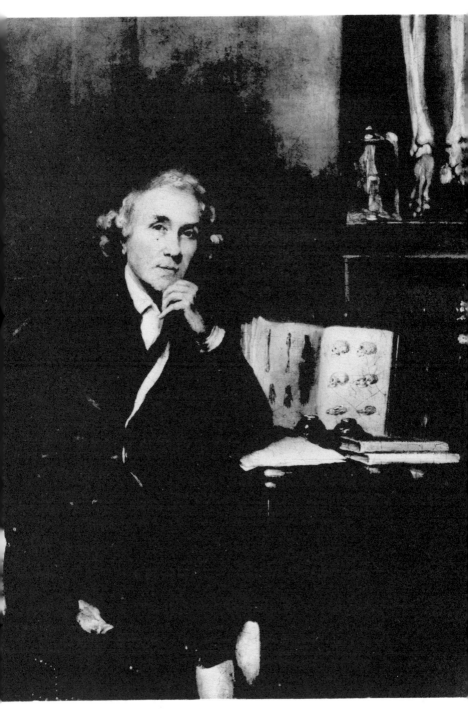

John Hunter
Portrait after Sir Joshua Reynolds

In July 1771, two months after he published the first part of his *Treatise on the Human Teeth*, John Hunter married a Miss Anne Home, who was the eldest daughter of Robert Home, a surgeon. Before her marriage, Miss Home had been well known for her lyrical poems, several of which, including 'My Mother bids me bind my Hair', had been set to music by Haydn. The two appear to have got on together reasonably well, though it is known that the new Mrs. Hunter's liking for fashionable society was in no way to her husband's taste. On one occasion, it is recorded, when he had found her drawing-room full of people of the type who liked to haunt literary 'salons', he told the guests that he 'had not been informed of this kick-up' and peremptorily ordered them to depart.

Just over a year after his marriage, John Hunter agreed that his wife's brother Everard Home should become one of his house pupils. The young man had been elected to Trinity College, Cambridge, but he resigned his scholarship as soon as he heard that the chance was open to him of studying under his celebrated brother-in-law. With Home to help him, John Hunter then started a historic series of lectures on the theory and practice of surgery – lectures in which, for the first time in Britain, truly scientific principles were enunciated on which the techniques of surgery could be firmly based. Only Hunter's house pupils and a few friends came to the earliest of these lectures, which were given on alternate evenings between October and April, but later his class grew until it included as many as thirty students, among them several men such as Astley Paston Cooper (born 1768) and Anthony Carlisle (born in the same year) who were later to become distinguished and influential surgeons. In spite of the importance of what he had to say, John Hunter never fully overcame his hatred of lecturing, and before he began to talk he was in the habit of taking large draughts of laudanum, to loosen his tongue.

From this time on, John Hunter's health was a constant source of anxiety to himself and to those around him, for

during the year in which he began his lectures he had his first
attack of angina pectoris, and he was always liable, afterwards, to suffer acute discomfort when he became emotion-
ally disturbed in any way. By 1777, he was suffering so
severely from vertigo that he decided to leave London
temporarily and to seek treatment at Bath. Edward Jenner
went to meet him there and, shocked by the altered
appearance of his former instructor, the Berkeley physician
formed the opinion, correctly, that Hunter was suffering
from an organic affection of the heart. Although he knew that
getting involved in any violent fuss or controversy might
well be fatal to him, John Hunter was quite unable to change
his cantankerous and provocative nature, and he was soon to
take a leading part in a famous quarrel.

The row was sparked off in January 1780 by a paper that
John read to the Royal Society on the structure of the human
placenta. In this paper, John asserted that he, and not his
brother William, had been the originator of certain important
discoveries about the circulation of the blood in the uterus
and the placenta. William, he said, had been claiming these
discoveries as his own both in his lectures and in his
published work. In a letter to the Society dated 3 February
1780, William retorted that the discoveries were well known
to be his and had never before been disputed. John countered
this by alleging that he had made the discoveries as far back as
May 1754, when he had been doing some dissection in
company with a Doctor Mackenzie. They had told William
about them, he said, but his elder brother had ridiculed their
ideas before adopting them, quietly, as his own. The officials
of the Royal Society decided that they would not print the
controversial paper or the acrimonious correspondence that
had followed it. There is little doubt that William was
justified in claiming credit for the discoveries that were made
in his own dissecting rooms and under his managerial
supervision, but John could not see the matter in that way
and the two brothers, after that, would have virtually
nothing to do with each other.

William's last years were saddened by gout, from which he suffered agonies. Late in March 1783, he insisted on giving his introductory lecture on the operations of surgery, though he had been ill for several days, and his associates had tried to persuade him to cancel this commitment. Towards the end of the lecture he fainted and had to be carried to bed. During the acute illness that followed, he observed to his friend Charles Combe (1743–1817) 'If I had strength enough to hold a pen, I would write how easy and pleasant a thing it is to die'. The end came on 30 March, and William Hunter was buried in St. James's Church, Piccadilly, in the Rector's vault. He left his museum to the care of three trustees, instructing them that after twenty years the entire contents should be given to the University of Glasgow.

In the year of his brother's death, John Hunter managed to add to his own museum the most extraordinary, and the most expensive, of all his acquisitions – he took possession of the body of O'Brien, or O'Byrne, the Irish giant. O'Brien, who was seven feet seven inches tall, had known for some time that the great Scottish surgeon intended to get his bones if he could, and he – O'Brien – had been determined to prevent this. The outsize Irishman had made a will in which he had ordered that after he had died the coffin that contained his body should be securely dropped into the sea in a very deep place. But John Hunter was quite equal to this: by bribing the undertaker with a large sum of money (one estimate was five hundred pounds, at that time quite a fortune) he ensured that O'Brien's body should be stolen while on its way to the sea. It arrived at the house in Earl's Court in John Hunter's own carriage and was immediately dissected and skeletonised.

In the same year, the lease expired of the house in Jermyn Street that had been William Hunter's before it became John's. Seeing that this was a good time to move, John Hunter bought, on twenty-four-year leases, two other houses. One was on the east side of Leicester Square, in which he intended to live, and the other in nearby Castle Street, in which house he intended to carry on his anatomical researches. Between the houses, there was a vacant plot of ground. During the next two or three years, Hunter built on this plot a large museum with lecture rooms beneath. When the museum was complete, Hunter moved his precious collections into it, with the able assistance of Everard Home and other members of his staff. Not everyone who applied to see John Hunter's museum would necessarily be admitted: the crusty old Scotsman was intensely conservative – he said that he wished that all the rascals who were dissatisfied with their country would leave it and he let it be known that he would rather see his museum on fire than have it shown to a democrat.

In 1785, John Hunter carried out one of his most important experiments – an experiment which was to result, in later decades, in a great saving of human lives. There were then, as now, large herds of fallow and red deer in Richmond Park. Hunter began by tying the artery that supplied blood to one of the antlers of one of the Park's bucks. Deprived of its blood supply, the antler became cold. That antler, it seemed, was doomed to die. Instead of dying, though, the antler regained, within a few days, its blood supply. This did not happen because Hunter had tied the artery carelessly, but because various subsidiary connecting arteries, above and below the ligature, had become enlarged and had started to do the work done formerly by the sealed blood vessel.

Next, Hunter had to turn this discovery to the benefit of his human patients. Up to that time, no doctor had known how to treat, satisfactorily, aneurisms – those pulsating swellings which are found in faulty arteries and which, if they are not dealt with properly, are liable to prove fatal. Usually, an early eighteenth-century surgeon would cut down through the superficial layers to such an aneurism and, after tying the artery above and below it, would remove its contents. This had, almost always, disastrous results. Occasionally, amputation of the affected limb would be preferred, in which case sepsis or shock, or sepsis and shock combined, would usually supervene.

In the following December, Hunter decided to tie the femoral artery of a patient who had an aneurism at the back of the leg. By tying the artery higher up, in a healthy part of the thigh, he was relying on the development of collateral circulation. The patient's limb would be in no undue danger of suffering from want of blood, he surmised. His confidence was justified: within six weeks, the patient was fully restored to health and was able to lead an active and useful life.

During the last eight years of John Hunter's life he was given many further honours. In 1786, he was appointed Deputy Surgeon General to the Army. After the death of Percivall Pott, two years later, he was regarded by all and sundry as the Head of the Surgical Profession. Two years after that, he was appointed Surgeon-General and Inspector-General of Hospitals. Busy as he was, he managed during those years to print, in his own house, and to publish important treatises on venereal disease (he is believed to have deliberately infected himself with syphilis during his researches into this sickness, which was very prevalent at the time) and on certain aspects of the animal economy. His *magnum opus* – the *Treatise on the Blood, Inflammation and Gunshot Wounds* – was still, as publishers say, 'in preparation'.

John Hunter's chance to finish this great work, which was to set the seal on his career, did not come until 1792, when Everard Home, who had been made Assistant Surgeon at St. George's Hospital, undertook to deliver Hunter's notes as a guide, so that Hunter could concentrate more effectively on his writing. At the same time, Mrs. Hunter received a letter from a school friend of hers who had married and was living in Cornwall. Could Mrs. Hunter's illustrious husband do with an apprentice? asked the friend. If so, the country lady went on, could she please recommend one of the local boys who made drawings with chalk on her floor? The friend's request was granted, and young William Clift, who came from a very poor family, was dispatched to London. He arrived in the capital on 14 February 1792. By a significant coincidence, it was both his own birthday and Doctor John

Hunter's. From that moment on, the young man seems to have devoted all his energies to serving John Hunter – drawing for him, dissecting for him, and helping him with his dearly-loved museum. In return for this selfless dedication, Clift was given an apprenticeship without being charged any fee.

Relieved by Everard Home and William Clift of so many of his usual chores, John Hunter should have been able to bring his great *Treatise* to a triumphant conclusion, but the famous anatomist was destined to die without seeing his most important publication through the press. His stubborn, outspoken nature was to be his undoing. He was, by this time, on thoroughly bad terms with most of the other surgeons connected with St. George's Hospital. The row came properly to the boil in 1792 when a new surgeon was to be elected to St. George's. John Hunter wanted Everard Home, his principal assistant, to be appointed. John Gunning, Master of the Surgeons' Company, was pressing the claims of Thomas Keate, his principal assistant. There was a short and bitter struggle between the rival factions. At the end of it, Gunning's man Keate got the job. John Hunter, predictably, was infuriated. He said he would no longer divide with the other St. George's Hospital surgeons the fees he received for instructing pupils, justifying this by claiming that the other surgeons did not do their part of the job properly. Equally furious, Gunning and his colleagues disputed Hunter's right to take this action, and the hospital's subscribers supported them.

The issue was to be resolved at a meeting of the Board to be held on 16 October 1793. On the morning of the – literally – fatal meeting, Hunter told his associates that he dreaded there being a serious dispute, as the excitement of any such conflict would, he knew, be extremely dangerous to him. His life, he used to say, was in the hands of any rascal who chose to annoy and tease him. He was not to be spared, however. While he was advancing his arguments he was rudely interrupted by one of the other surgeons present, probably

Gunning. The shock was too much for Hunter, who immediately stopped speaking and withdrew into an adjoining room. There he collapsed into the arms of a Doctor Robinson, physician to the hospital, and within a few seconds he was dead. An autopsy was to confirm Edward Jenner's diagnosis – the great man's mitral valves and coronary arteries were extensively ossified and there were other indications of serious heart disease.

Although it is true that John Hunter was dead before the nineteenth century started, his influence on practitioners and students of medicine and surgery was as powerful as if he were alive. His museum contained more than thirteen thousand specimens. Many of these were unique, and the collection was supplemented by numerous volumes of manuscript notes which had been compiled by Hunter, and which described, in the greatest detail, the exhibits. Everard Home, appointed joint executor with a Doctor Baillie of Hunter's last will and testament, was faced with an enormous problem: what shoud he do with all those specimens? For a start, he engaged William Clift and employed him to take care, temporarily, of the collection, paying him, for doing this, only a few shillings a week.

Then Home and Baillie offered to sell the collection to the British Government. William Pitt, who was Prime Minister at the time, did not take kindly to the idea. 'What? buy preparations?' he is said to have exploded. 'Why, I have not money enough to purchase gunpowder!' In spite of Pitt's initial reaction, Hunter's treasures were eventually acquired by the State and given, as a Trust, to the College of Surgeons. The Surgeons took William Clift into their own employment, increased his salary to £100 per year, and gave him the grand-sounding title of 'Conservator' of the Museum. Having supervised two major moves of the collection – the first to a temporary store, the second to its new and permanent home – without the loss or damage of a single specimen, Clift then devoted himself for more than half a century to the enlargement and enrichment of the Museum and to the proper display and illustration of its contents. Students of comparative anatomy and physiology, during this critical period, were almost without exception deeply indebted to Clift.

Shortly before John Hunter's collection was due to be delivered to the College of Surgeons in 1800, Everard Home instructed William Clift to deliver John Hunter's notes to Home's own house. Home was going to produce and get published a scholarly edition of these notes that could be regarded as the Official Catalogue of the Museum, or so he said, and immensely valuable such a work would have been, too. But the years rolled on without the appearance of the Great Official Catalogue. The Surgeons kept urging Everard Home to complete it, as he had promised, and they offered to provide him with assistance, but their offers of help were consistently rejected. By 1818 Home, by that time a baronet, had managed to produce only a synopsis of the projected Catalogue, though he had meanwhile been using Hunter's notes for the preparation of numerous papers that he had been delivering, as if they were all his own unaided work, to the members of the Royal Society.

In July 1823 came the *dénouement*, when Home confessed to Clift that he had just burned all John Hunter's papers, almost setting fire to his own house in the process. Hunter, when dying, had asked him to destroy the papers, Home claimed, but this is unlikely to have been true, for if it were, why should Home have kept them and made use of them for his own purposes for nearly thirty years, before carrying out the dead man's wishes?

Clift, understandably, was deeply shocked by Home's revelation. 'Well, Sir Everard, there is but one more thing to be done, and that is to destroy the Collection', he moaned, and burst into tears.

The Collection continued to be used for example and instruction until it was partly destroyed by aerial bombardment on the night of 10 May 1941.

# 3

# Some Contemporaries and Followers of the Hunters

*. . . Long is the way*
*And hard, that out of hell leads up to light . . .*

JOHN MILTON, 1608–74, *Paradise Lost*

The compelling influence of John Hunter was to be quickly felt in most parts of the civilised world. The message was to be carried to America, in the first place, by the family Hewson.

William Hunter engaged as an assistant, it will be recalled, a young man named William Hewson. Hewson had travelled to London from Hexham in Northumberland, in 1759, to study at Guy's and St Thomas's Hospitals, and he had lodged with John Hunter while he was attending William Hunter's lectures on anatomy. When John Hunter left William Hunter in 1760 and set off with the expedition to Belle Île, Hewson had seemed an ideal person to take John Hunter's place as an instructor in the dissecting rooms in Lichfield Street. Hewson got on with William very well, and in 1761 the older man said that he would take him into partnership as long as Hewson would agree to study first, at Edinburgh. Hewson accepted this offer. In the autumn of 1762 he returned to London from Scotland and started to share the duties and the profits of William Hunter's consistently successful school.

Hewson was a brilliant anatomist and researcher. He was particularly successful in matters concerning the coagulation of the blood and he managed to isolate a key protein in the coagulation process – 'fibrinogen', which he called 'coagulable lymph'. He also investigated the lymphatic system and described the red blood cells. In 1770, however, Hewson decided to get married to a Miss Mary Stevenson, in whose mother's house the eminent American Benjamin Franklin had been lodging since he first arrived in London in 1757. The pair set up house on their own, but Hewson's removal from William Hunter's establishment did not please the great obstetrician and Hunter made this an excuse for breaking off his partnership with Hewson. This was a great blow to the younger man, for he knew that he would no longer be welcome in the anatomical school which was entirely William Hunter's property. During the twelve months which had to elapse, according to the terms of their contract, before the dissolution of the partnership was complete, Hewson started to collect specimens for an anatomical museum of his own. He had a lecture theatre built adjoining his new home, and he began to prepare a course of lectures. In September 1772 he started lecturing on his own account and he kept this up for nearly two years, attracting large numbers of hearers by the extent of his knowledge and the brilliance of his delivery.

Early in the summer of 1774, Hewson injured himself slightly while he was making a dissection, and serious symptoms soon appeared. After a few days' illness, during which all too little could be done to relieve his condition, he died, leaving a widow who had two young children and was expecting a third. Advised by Benjamin Franklin, the widow decided to emigrate to America. Her second son – Thomas Tickell Hewson – studied medicine at Edinburgh before becoming a distinguished physician. He was made, eventually, President of the College of Physicians at Philadelphia, and he advocated there the methods his father had learned in the school of the Hunters.

John Syng Physick (1768–1837) has often been called 'The Father of American Surgery'. After attending a course of John Hunter's London lectures, Physick was urged by Hunter to remain in London and to act as his assistant, but he preferred to return to his native country. Unfortunately for Physick, a serious epidemic of yellow fever broke out almost immediately after he had started to practise.

He worked intensively for a time in his attempts to alleviate the sufferings of his stricken patients. Then he caught the fever himself and nearly died. He recovered eventually, but he never fully regained his original vigour.[1] In spite of this, he soon became noted for his excellence as a surgeon, being appointed Surgeon to the Pennsylvania Hospital and Professor of Surgery at the University. Like John Hunter, Physick was reluctant to use the knife in cases that could be dealt with by any other form of treatment, reserving operative surgery, in the main, for such well-tried processes as lithotomy and the removal of cataracts.[2]

Three of John Hunter's pupils who stayed in Britain made international reputations for themselves in differing ways.

The work done by Edward Jenner has been described in detail elsewhere.[3] By 1800, members of the medical profession, in London, were gradually becoming aware of Jenner's seventy-five-page-long pamphlet *An Inquiry into the Cause and Effects of the Variolae Vaccinae, a Disease discovered in some of the Western Counties of England, particularly Gloucestershire, and known by the name of the Cowpox*. The significance of the last words of the pamphlet – 'the cowpox protects the human constitution from the infection of smallpox' – was belatedly being realised. There were those, like a Doctor Ingenhousz, who were disputing the validity of Jenner's conclusions, but the Gloucestershire physician was replying patiently to the more vociferous objectors. Meanwhile, he was obtaining as much good, reliable lymph as he could and sending it away.

From time to time, Jenner's quiet but persistent campaign met with sudden and sensational setbacks – as, for example, when lymph from smallpox pustules was used by inexperienced practitioners instead of cowpox lymph, which helped, of course, to spread the disease instead of checking it. But news of his great discovery had started to travel abroad – to France, Spain, and other European countries, and to America, where an account of Jenner's experiments with the cowpox was sent to the *Columbian Sentinel* by Doctor Benjamin Waterhouse, Professor of Physic at Cambridge,

Massachusetts. It was printed under the ambiguous heading 'Something Curious in the Medical Line'. Certain that he had a public duty to experiment, himself, with the new technique, Doctor Waterhouse wrote to England asking that some of the cowpox matter might be sent to him for trial. After several unsuccessful attempts had been made to send active lymph over the Atlantic, Jenner managed to get some to Doctor Waterhouse 'by a short passage from Bristol', and with this the Cambridge professor inoculated all the younger members of his family.

By 1801, all the sailors of the British fleet were being vaccinated. The medical officers of the fleet, in that year, gave Jenner a special gold medal to demonstrate their appreciation of his efforts. Numerous congratulatory addresses that arrived at Berkeley from that time on showed that vaccination was known and was being recommended by doctors in most parts of the civilised world. The Empress of Russia sent Jenner a ring and the Gentry of Gloucestershire gave him a service of plate, and various other honours were heaped on him.

But the Gloucestershire doctor had suffered financially by being morally obliged to spend so much time on work of a scientific and entirely unpaid nature, and eventually a comittee was appointed by Parliament to consider this. 'If Doctor Jenner had not chosen openly and honourably to explain to the public all he knew upon the subject he might have acquired a considerable fortune. In my opinion it is the most important discovery ever made in medicine', reported Doctor Matthew Baillie, executor of the late Doctor John Hunter. After the committee had reported to Parliament on 2 June 1802, Jenner was granted the sum of £10,000, and this was later doubled. A 'Jennerian Institution' set up in London for the promotion of vaccination and 'the extermination of the smallpox' was replaced, with Government aid, in 1808, by the National Vaccine Establishment. Smallpox, from that time on, was a rapidly diminishing terror.

John Abernethy was born in London in 1764. His father

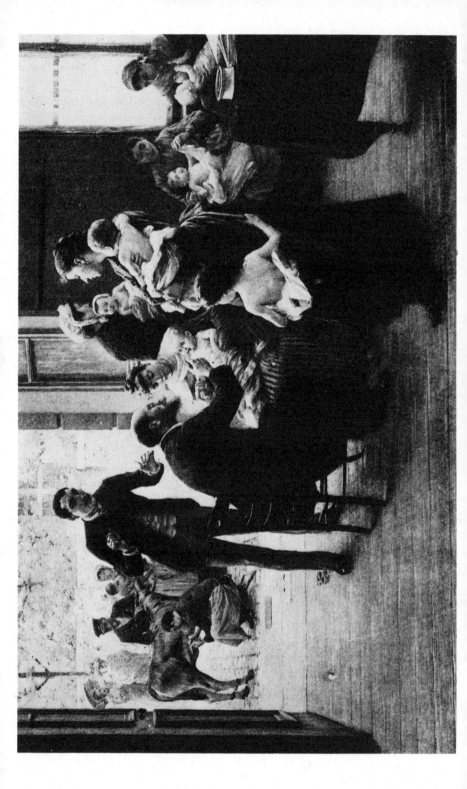

was an Irish merchant of Scottish extraction. When he was fifteen years old, Abernethy was taken on as an apprentice by a Mr Blicke, who was at that time Surgeon to St Bartholomew's Hospital. Eight years later, Abernethy was appointed Assistant Surgeon to St Bartholomew's Hospital – a post he was to hold for more than a quarter of a century. Soon after he was promoted, Abernethy began to give lectures on anatomy at his house in Bartholomew Close, near the hospital. These lectures, given with great clarity and a pronounced sense of drama, attracted a large number of students – so many, that the Governors of the hospital decided that they ought to build a lecture theatre in which Abernethy could lecture on anatomy, physiology and surgery. This is usually regarded as the beginning of the School of Medicine at St Bartholomew's. But Abernethy's lectures were by no means original – he was, himself, a regular attender at John Hunter's classes and was accustomed to having private discussions with the great man on topics of particular medical interest. So the ideas spread by the disciple were, in the first place, largely those of the Master.

While he was still under the influence of John Hunter, Abernethy caused a minor sensation in medical circles by carrying Hunter's operation for the cure of aneurism a stage further: he tied successfully a patient's iliac artery. As a man, he was exceptionally blunt and overbearing and the brusque way in which he treated the patients who flocked to his consulting rooms became, eventually, notorious. To one over-fed, under-exercised Alderman the advice he gave was 'Live on sixpence a day, and earn it'. Another patient who was a hypochondriac was advised by Abernethy to travel to Inverness to consult a certain 'Doctor Robinson'. This 'Doctor Robinson' was a figment of Abernethy's fancy, but the long and worrying journey to Scotland and the anger felt by the patient as he returned took the man's mind effectively off his imagined ills and may have brought about a cure. At any rate, Abernethy was relieved of one of his most importunate patients by this ruse.[4]

As Abernethy aged, he lost much of his enthusiasm for operating, and indeed in later life he could hardly be induced to take up the knife. His ideas became set, too. For instance, he believed firmly that virtually all human diseases that were not the immediate consequence of some accidental injury would be found to be caused by some disorder of the digestive system. This being so, all such diseases could be cured, he insisted, by careful attention to the diet, by small doses of calomel, or mercuric sulphide, and by such well-tried purgatives as the 'blue pill'. Abernethy's system was based on a gross over-simplification, but it did lead many of his contemporaries to study the general health of their patients and in that sense he may be said to have introduced a new principle into British medical practice.

Astley Paston Cooper – the third of these eminent pupils of John Hunter – was born in 1768, and was the fourth son of the Reverend Samuel Cooper, D.D., curate of Great Yarmouth. Astley Cooper was apprenticed at an early age to his grandfather, who was a surgeon of some note and settled in Norwich. Next, Astley went to Henry Cline, Surgeon at St Thomas's Hospital, who taught him wisely and thoroughly and encouraged him to attend Hunter's lectures. Then, in 1791, Cline appointed Astley Cooper to be joint Lecturer with himself in anatomy and surgery, and in the same year Astley Cooper married a Miss Anne Cock, who brought him a considerable fortune.

In 1793, Astley Cooper was selected to lecture on anatomy at the College of Surgeons, and seven years later he was appointed Surgeon to Guy's Hospital. A Mr Travers, who became Cooper's articled pupil at that time, recorded that Cooper had the handsomest, most intelligent and finely formed countenance he had ever seen, and that he moved with grace, vigour and elasticity. His charm, his markedly pleasing manners, his excellent memory and his exceptional power of inspiring confidence in patients and students alike combined to make him a paragon of the times. By 1806 he had built up an extensive private practice and for some years

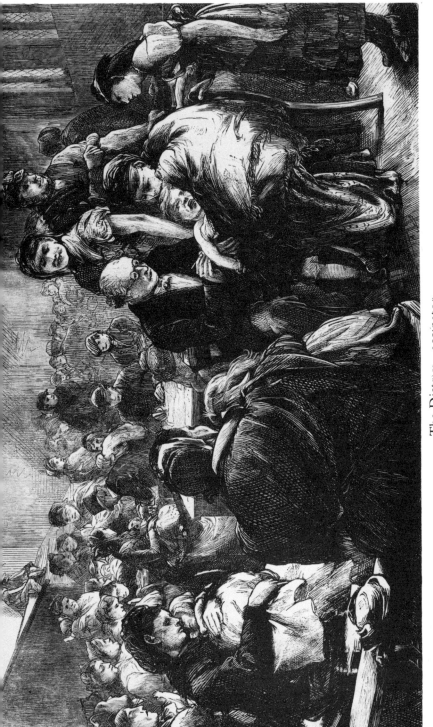

The District vaccinator

after that his annual income exceeded by far that earned by the Prime Minister. His largest fee – a thousand guineas – was passed to him by a wealthy West Indian planter named Hyatt, in Mr Hyatt's nightcap, after he had successfully operated on Mr Hyatt for the stone.[4] Cooper's servant – a man named Charles – was said to earn himself several hundred pounds every year 'on the side' by showing patients into the great man's consulting room out of their proper turn.[5] In 1820, Astley Cooper was asked to carry out a small operation on King George IV, for the removal of a sebaceous cyst on the head. The operation was once again entirely successful, and Astley Cooper was rewarded with a baronetcy.

Five years after that, Sir Astley Cooper gave up the post of Lecturer in Anatomy at St Thomas's Hospital, taking it for granted that he would be succeeded by his nephew, Bransby Cooper. But he was wrong – a Mr South was appointed instead. In high dudgeon, Sir Astley then persuaded Mr Harrison, the Treasurer of Guy's Hospital, to found a separate medical school at Guy's so that his nephew could be its Lecturer in Anatomy. The Governors of St Thomas's retaliated by refusing to allow Sir Astley to remove the valuable specimens that he had left there as the visual aids for his lectures. Piqued further by this, Sir Astley then set out to assemble an entirely new collection for the benefit of the students at Guy's. The successful launching of this famous medical school was due, in no small measure, to Sir Astley's vigour and enterprise.[6]

The Napoleonic Wars cut off nearly all channels of communication between the leaders of medical and surgical research in Britain and their contemporaries in Europe. When the wars were over, the news that filtered through from France and her Allies proved to be of some importance. In 1808, for instance, Jean Nicholas Corvisart (born 1755), who was Napoleon Bonaparte's personal physician and friend, had found a little book. Written by one Leopold Auenbrugger, it was only 95 pages long, and had been published in 1761. It had been read for a few months by those who might be professionally interested and its contents had been considered of little importance. For nearly fifty years it had been completely forgotten. As Corvisart studied this little treatise, he saw clearly that the author's discoveries were of real diagnostic significance. So, he set to work to translate the pamphlet from Latin into French.

Auenbrugger had been born in 1722. He was the son of a man who kept an inn at Graz, in Austria. During his boyhood, he had noticed that his father would tap on the side of a wine barrel if he wished to estimate how much wine that barrel still contained: the sound produced by the knock, echoing in the void at the top of the barrel, would tell Auenbrugger the elder, with his experienced ear, just what he needed to know. When Auenbrugger the younger had finished his medical training and had been appointed physician to the Military Hospital of Vienna, he remembered the barrel-tapping at Graz, and he tried to apply the same principle to the examination of the human thorax. His experiments were successful. So his *Inventum Novum* began with the words 'I here present the reader with a new sign that I have discovered for detecting disease of the chest'. Thousands of copies of Corvisart's translation of Auenbrugger's treatise were sold, and the techniques that the Graz innkeeper's son had recommended were quickly adopted by doctors in most of the countries of Europe.[7]

Eleven years after Corvisart's Auenbrugger appeared, another French doctor – René Théophile Hyacinthe Laënnec – had made an equally valuable contribution to medical techniques. Laënnec had been born in 1781 at Quimper, in Brittany. After his medical training he had been appointed physician to the Necker Hospital in Paris. Shortly after he took up this post, he was required to examine an exceptionally stout patient – a man who was so fat that Laënnec found it difficult to listen to the sounds of his heart by the ear-to-chest method used, probably, since the days of Hippocrates. Inspired, it is believed, by having seen two children playing with a log of wood – one of the children had tapped one end of the log, while the other had listened, at the other end, to the sounds produced – Laënnec took a sheet of paper, rolled it up so that it formed a tube and, putting one end to his patient's chest and the other to his own ear, discovered that he could hear the heart's action 'in a manner more clear and distinct than I had ever been able to do by the immediate application of the ear'.[8]

Three years after that, Laënnec made his great discovery known to the medical profession in a book that he called *Traité de l'Auscultation Médiate*. The older method of 'auscultation', or chest listening, had been not only ineffective, he suggested, but it had been inconvenient, indelicate, and, in hospitals, even disgusting![9] Instead, he proposed the use of a 'stethoscope' or 'cylinder of wood an inch and a half in diameter and a foot long, perforated by a bore three lines wide and hollowed out into funnel shape at one of its extremities'. With such a stethoscope, he claimed, one could hear sounds that had never been heard before. He used a number of ingenious new words such as aegophony and pectoriloquy in an attempt to differentiate between these sounds. The book caused a minor sensation in medical circles in Paris and was soon published in other countries besides France. In the second edition, Laënnec added detailed descriptions of the diseases of the chest that had been identified up to that time, and the enlarged book was for a long time regarded as a classic.

But Laënnec, unfortunately, was himself suffering from a disease of the lungs, and the labours involved in the production of his stethoscopes and the writing of his book had totally exhausted him. He retired to Brittany in a vain attempt to regain his health. By 1822 he had recovered sufficiently to be able to accept the Chair of Medicine in the College of France, but there was little hope that he could sustain the appointment for long, and he died four years later – by a cruel irony, the victim of the disease, pulmonary tuberculosis, that he had done so much to explain. His treatise was translated into English by John Forbes and published in 1821, and his methods were quickly adopted by the members of the go-ahead Dublin School of Medicine after their leader William Stokes (born 1804) had fully appreciated the use of the stethoscope. In America, the improved methods of physical diagnosis that had been developed in Europe were recommended chiefly by a group of young Boston doctors who had been to Paris for their postgraduate training.

# 4

# Body Snatchers

It was quite right and proper for William and John Hunter to suggest that their pupils and their pupils' pupils should base their surgical and medical practice on an exact knowledge of anatomy. There was, however, at the start of the nineteenth century an almost insurmountable obstacle: bodies that could legally be dissected were in regrettably short supply.

The laws that dealt with the disposal of corpses – or 'subjects', as cadavers were euphemistically called by dissectors and potential dissectors – were unhelpful, to say the least. As far back as the reign of King Henry VIII, it had been decided that the members of the Company of Barbers and Surgeons should have, as by right, the bodies of those malefactors who had suffered public execution. Then in 1752 instructions were given that the bodies of murderers executed in London and Middlesex 'should be conveyed to the hall of the Surgeons' Company to be dissected and anatomised.' With dissection regarded as the proper and fitting end for the eternally damned, it was hardly surprising that members of the public were generally reluctant to hand over the bodies of their dead relatives to suffer the ultimate shame.

With anatomists inspired by the Hunters seeking bodies for research purposes in ever-increasing numbers and the officials of the Surgeons' Company insisting that their members should have some knowledge at least of anatomy before they started to cut into living flesh, a serious shortage of 'subjects' was bound to develop. As a result of the inadequacy of the law, an illicit traffic in dead bodies grew up.

The business was conducted, mainly, by the callous operators known as 'body-snatchers' or 'resurrection men'. These agents might be the relatively few 'regular men', who had no other reliable source of income, or they might be the 'outsiders', or part-time operatives, who needed to do a quiet bit of body-snatching when money was short.

In the ordinary way of business, the body-snatchers relied on robbing newly-filled graves, bribing the graveyard attendant, or attendants, if necessary, so that he, or they, would be looking the other way as the paymasters went about their gruesome work. The rivalry between the different firms, or syndicates, of resurrection men became keen, however, and the 'snatchers' had to go to extraordinary lengths to get hold of the bodies they needed, before their rivals got hold of them. The rougher men would deal violently with their competitors.

Sometimes, the professional body-snatchers would pretend that they were the relatives of a person who had recently died, so that they could decently and reverently remove, from a hospital or parish workhouse, the body they wanted to sell. Really swift-thinking body-snatchers were even known to take a corpse that was already on the dissecting table, claiming it as theirs so that they could carry it away and sell it somewhere else.

Virtually every surgeon and private teacher of anatomy had to come to some kind of financial arrangement, at one point at least in his career, with the body-snatchers. Even a most distinguished figure in the medical profession might have to commission one or more of the rogues to retrieve for him the body of a patient who had undergone some unusually interesting operation, or who had died from some disease that would make the outcome of an autopsy especially instructive. So, the cost of a 'subject' rose, at one time, to as much as fifteen guineas – then a very considerable sum – and, as well as this, the anatomy instructors would have to pay the gang-leaders 'opening money' at the start of each course of lectures, so that they could rely on a regular supply of cadavers. Some of the gang-leaders even charged 'retaining fees' while the anatomy students were on vacation. They would demand financial compensation, too, if any members of their gangs were unlucky enough to get apprehended and sent to prison.

As the prices charged for cadavers soared, more and more medical men began to resent the body-snatchers' extortionate demands, and a few of the dissectors even tried to form an 'Anatomy Club' in a vain attempt to control the level of payment. The Resurrectionists retaliated by playing some humiliating tricks on the professional men who were attempting to limit their livelihood. A Mr Joshua Brookes of Great Marlborough Street, for instance, who had made himself particularly objectionable to the members of the fraternity was punished by having badly decomposed bodies deposited on his doorstep. And once, this Mr Brookes was actually persuaded to buy a 'body', done up in a sack, that turned out to be a live member of the gang of snatchers with whom he was particularly at loggerheads.

By the beginning of the nineteenth century, a few forward-looking people had realised that some rational system would have to be devised, and quickly, for the alternative disposal of human remains.

As far back as 1769, when he came of age, Jeremy Bentham, who was to become the great utilitarian philosopher and the country's leading writer on jurisprudence, had taken some preliminary steps in that direction. He had been a weakly and undersized child and, during his minority, he had given a lot of thought to the needs of doctors. As soon as he was legally able to do so, Bentham made a will in which he requested that his body, when he eventually died, should be dissected for the benefit of mankind. In spite of the general ill-health he had suffered in his youth, Bentham managed to stay alive, and surprisingly robust, until the year 1832. When seriously ill, Bentham asked his doctor to tell him if there were any chance that he might recover. The doctor told him that there was no chance at all of that happening, and Bentham replied serenely, 'Very well, be it so. Then minimise pain'. According to his wishes, shortly after, Bentham's body was dissected. Dressed in his usual clothes, his skeleton is preserved, still, in a glass-fronted case at University College, London.

Body-snatching had been very much in the public eye during the last years of Jeremy Bentham's life, and feeling on the subject had reached a new pitch of intensity. Tough guards were being specially appointed to watch over recent graves, and these men were frequently coming into conflict with the body-snatchers, some of whom they violently man-handled. The members of the Government were slow to take any positive action. They knew that the medical profession's need for subjects was urgent, but they knew, too, that the current outcry would make satisfactory legislation on the subject difficult to frame, and probably almost impossible to pass. In an attempt to ride the storm, they set up a Select Committee on Anatomy. At the meetings of this committee many distinguished medical men gave evidence, and so, too, did some of the body-snatchers, though the latter were allowed to appear in an anonymous capacity. In the statement he gave to the Committee, Sir Astley Cooper alleged:

The Law does not prevent our obtaining the body of an individual if we think proper; for there is no person, let his situation in life be what it may, whom, if I were disposed to dissect, I could not obtain . . . The Law only enhances the price and does not prevent the exhumation.

The Select Committee presented its report to Parliament in 1828, and, as happens so often, there the matter might have been allowed to rest. In this instance, though, the Govern-ment was forced to take action by the deeds of some particularly ruthless criminals – one gang of them in Edinburgh, the other in the East End of London.

The Edinburgh ghouls were based in a squalid lodging

house – 'Log's' – that was situated in one of the poorest quarters of the city. Mrs Log, widow of the lodging house's keeper, had married a rough Irish labourer called William Hare, and he and one of his cronies named William Burke were the principal malefactors. Aware that the professional body-snatchers in their neighbourhood had plenty of money to spend on gin and the other necessities of life, Burke and Hare took the body of an old pauper who had died at Log's to the back door of an anatomy school run by the brilliant lecturer Doctor Knox, and were given good money for it – more, by far, than they could have earned in several weeks in their normal occupations. They returned to the school a few days later with another body, and were given more money. They became Doctor Knox's main source of supply.

The later bodies provided by William Burke and William Hare for the use of the students at Doctor Knox's Academy of Anatomy were not, however, as straightforwardly acquired as the body of the first old pauper had been. The later cadavers were 'produced' for sale by a relatively simple expedient: unsuspecting people were lured to Log's Lodging House, made drunk with rum or whisky, and then held down on a rough bed by Hare while Burke, kneeling on their chests, literally pressed the life out of them.

Nobody knows, or will ever know, exactly how many living people were quickly and callously converted into saleable anatomical subjects by Burke and Hare, aided and abetted by their womenfolk. It is certain, though, that the number of their victims ran into double figures. The members of the gang continued their successful careers until a female lodger, whom they had turned out of the lodging house so that they could carry out undisturbed another murder, returned before they had had a chance to carry off the body to Doctor Knox's. She found the cadaver hidden in a pile of straw, and raised the alarm. The men and their women were promptly arrested.

Burke was convicted on the testimony of Hare, who was persuaded to turn King's Evidence, and was publicly hanged before a large crowd in the streets of Edinburgh. Hare should have been released from prison, according to the agreement which was normally reached with those who gave evidence for the Crown against their confederates, but it was known that the people of Edinburgh were waiting for him so that they could deal with him themselves. His prison cell had to become a sanctuary. When Hare was smuggled out of the prison, late at night, after more than a month had elapsed, in a carriage which had its blinds drawn tightly down, the mob was waiting for him. He was thrown into a convenient lime pit. He is said to have earned some kind of living, after that, as a blind beggar plying his trade in Oxford Street, London. Doctor Knox, driven from Edinburgh by the scandal that ensued, was also forced to move south. He settled in London's East End.

Some, at least, of the criminals who provided the London teaching hospitals with the bodies they needed were as enterprising as Burke and Hare. The gruesome nature of the activities of one particularly evil group of men, based on the East End, came to light in 1831.

Suspicion was aroused when two of the men – John Bishop and James May – paid a visit, by way of doing business, to the dissecting rooms of King's College, London. There, May asked the porter whether he 'wanted anything', meaning, in the language of those who specialised in the ancient East End craft of body-snatching (as the *Newgate Calendar* put it), whether he wanted to buy a subject. When Mr Partridge, the anatomical demonstrator, told them that nine guineas was the greatest amount he would pay, the two men went away and returned, later, with two other men, Thomas Williams and James Shields, who were carrying a hamper. The hamper contained the body of a boy who had been about fourteen years old. Thinking that the body looked particularly fresh, the porter asked the men what the boy had died of. May, who had had a lot to drink, answered that that was no business of theirs, or his either. So, the porter told the anatomical demonstrator that he was uneasy about the body.

The demonstrator noticed that the body appeared not to have been buried, and that it had a cut on its forehead, so he felt a little uneasy about it, too. Members of the recently formed Metropolitan Police were called, and the four men were taken into custody.

It was soon established that the prisoners Bishop, May and Williams were frequenters of a noted house-of-call for body-snatchers – the 'Fortune of War' public house, in Smithfield – and, on the day before their arrest, May had been observed there with a number of human teeth in a handkerchief. The teeth had had some portions of the flesh of the gum still adhering to them, and May had been seen pouring water on them in order to clean it away. A few hours later, Shields had joined them, and Bishop had gone off to fetch a hamper from St Bartholomew's Hospital. Having heard this evidence, the magistrate remanded the men in custody.

Next day, the police went to Bishop's house in Nova Scotia Gardens, Bethnal Green, and searched the premises thoroughly. Buried in the garden, they found various items of clothing that had been taken off a number of 'subjects' for which two at least of the men in custody had obtained ready money.

The trial of the prisoners Bishop, May and Williams upon the charge of murder took place on Friday 2 December 1831. At ten o'clock precisely, Chief Justice Tindal, Mr Justice Littledale and Mr Baron Vaughan took their seats upon the bench, 'the remaining portion of which was instantly occupied by members of the nobility and persons of distinction, among whom was His Royal Highness the Duke of Sussex'. All three men were found guilty. The verdict was received in Court 'with becoming silence; but the moment it was conveyed to the immense multitude assembled outside they evinced their satisfaction at the result by loud and long-continued cheering and clapping of hands'. The noise was so deafening that the windows of the Court had to be closed in order that the voice of the Recorder might be heard as he passed the sentence of death.

Before he was hanged, with Williams, outside Newgate Prison, in the presence of thirty thousand spectators, John Bishop was persuaded to make a confession:

I, John Bishop, do hereby declare and confess that the boy . . . was a Lincolnshire boy. I and Williams took him to my house about half-past ten o'clock on Thursday night, the 3rd November, from the Bell in Smithfield. We lighted a candle, and gave the boy some bread and cheese; and after he had eaten, we gave him a cup full of rum, with about half a small phial of laudanum in it. I had bought the rum the same evening in Smithfield, and the laudanum also in small quantities at different shops. There was no water or other liquid put into the cup with the rum and laudanum. The boy drank the contents of the cup directly, in two draughts, and afterwards a little beer. In about ten minutes he fell asleep in the chair on which he sat, and I removed him from the chair to the floor and laid him on his side. We then went out and left him there. We had a quartern of gin and a pint of beer at the Feathers, near Shoreditch church, and then went home again, having been away from the boy about twenty minutes. We found him asleep as we had left him. We took him directly, asleep and insensible, into the garden, and tied a cord to his feet, to enable us to pull him up by; and I then took him in my arms and let him slide from them headlong into the well in the garden; whilst Williams held the cord to prevent the boy going altogether too low in the well. He was nearly wholly in the water, his feet being just above the surface. Williams fastened the other end of the cord round the paling, to prevent the body getting beyond our reach. The boy struggled a little with his arms and legs in the water, and the water bubbled a minute. We waited till these symptoms were past, and then went indoors, and afterwards I think we went out and walked down Shoreditch to occupy the time; and in three-quarters of an hour we returned, and took him out of the well, by pulling him by the cord attached to his feet.[1]

After describing two more murders carried out by the same technique which, he claimed, allowed the mixtures of rum and laudanum to run out of the bodies at the mouth, Bishop finished:

> I have followed the course of obtaining a livelihood as a body-snatcher for twelve years, and have obtained and sold, I think, from five hundred to a thousand bodies; but I declare before God that they were all obtained after death, and that, with the above exceptions, I am ignorant of any murder for that or any other purpose.[2]

A few months after Bishop and Williams were executed – four years, that is, after the Select Committee on Anatomy had presented its Report to Parliament – a revolutionary Anatomy Act was put on the Statute Book, its passage through the House of Commons and the House of Lords having been undoubtedly speeded by the recent *causes célèbres*.

By this Act, the Government swept entirely away the practice by which the bodies of murderers were handed over to the surgeons for dissection. No longer would the old stigma be attached to being dissected. The Act laid down that properly authenticated certificates should be issued after every death, and that the bodies should afterwards be decently buried; it ensured that properly qualified doctors, teachers and students should be granted licences which would allow them legally to practise dissection; and it stipulated that any legally appointed executor or any other person who had lawful possession of a body could give it up for dissection as long as no relative of the deceased raised any objection.

The Anatomy Act of 1832 was wholly successful. After it became law, a sufficient supply of cadavers was always available in Britain. The 'Resurrection Men' were driven out of business, in consequence, and the bodies of those who had not wished to submit to the anatomists were allowed to lie quietly in their graves.

# 5

# *Anaesthetics*

*. . . Give me to drink mandragora*
*That I might sleep out this great gap of time*
*My Antony is away . . .*

WILLIAM SHAKESPEARE, *Antony and Cleopatra*

*. . . Care-charming Sleep, thou easer of all woes,*
*Brother to Death . . .*

FRANCIS BEAUMONT (1584–1616)
and
JOHN FLETCHER (1579–1625)
*Valentinian*, Act 5

Until the nineteenth century, men and women had to face the agonies of surgery, when this was necessary, without any reliable form of relief. As far back as the first century A.D., Dioscorides, in his *Herbal*, was advocating that the wine made from the bark of the mandrake root should be given to patients who were about to be cut or cauterised. They would then be unable to feel pain, he added, since they would be overcome by 'dead sleep'. Substances used for the relief of pain during the Middle Ages included opium and cannabis indica, and alcohol was administered to many patients so that they would be stupefied, if not actually unconscious, while they were undergoing essential surgery. A variety of other pain-killing techniques was employed. Some medical men believed that they could reduce suffering by applying pressure to nerves; others tried to freeze the part of the patient's body that was to be operated on, and there were a number of practitioners who even went as far as trying asphyxiation. In the mid-eighteenth century, hypnotism of a sort was advocated by Franz Anton Mesmer, but the commission of scientists and physicians appointed by the French Government to investigate his activities was not enthusiastic, and the poor man was driven from his flourishing practice to a life of obscurity in Switzerland.

The first really important steps towards the conquest of pain were taken by Humphry Davy. Davy was born at Penzance, in Cornwall, on 17 December 1778. He was the son of a gentleman of means who amused himself, principally, by wood carving and other cultural activities. At an early age, Humphry was sent to the Penzance Grammar School, and there – according to contemporary records – he quickly showed that he was an unusually gifted boy. When he was only eight years old he would collect together a small crowd of other boys and, standing on a cart in the market place of the town, he would lecture to them on the subject of his recent studies. The applause of his companions was his recompense, he said, for any punishments he might be awarded for being idle.

Davy became interested in experimental science while he was still only a boy. The man who aroused this interest – Robert Dunkin – was a member of the Society of Friends, who earned a living as a saddler, but who spent most of his spare time constructing electrical machines, Voltaic piles, Leyden jars and other items of scientific equipment, and devising models that would illustrate the rudiments of mechanics. From the school at Penzance, Davy was sent in 1793 to Truro, to finish his education under a Reverend Doctor Cardew, who does not seem to have put any undue pressure on him. 'I consider it fortunate I was left so much to myself as a child and put upon no particular plan of study', Davy commented later. 'What I am, I made myself.'

In 1794, Davy's father died, and at the suggestion of John Tonkin, an old family friend who was an eminent surgeon at Penzance, the lad was then apprenticed to John Bingham Borlase, a surgeon who had a large practice in the town. This suited young Davy very well, for there was a large attic under the roof of John Tonkin's house, and here Davy was able to carry out his first independent chemical experiments, while his friends said they were afraid that he would blow them all into the air and his eldest sister complained of the damage done to her dresses by the corrosive substances that Humphry was using in his 'laboratory'.

Davy's career was given a further fortuitous boost when he happened to be swinging on the half-gate of the house of the surgeon to whom he had been apprenticed. By chance, a distinguished scholar named Davies Giddy happened to be passing – Giddy had been High Sheriff of Cornwall in two of the years that had recently passed, and he had many influential friends among the scientists of London and the Universities of Oxford and Cambridge. Seeing the youth swinging on the gate, Giddy stopped and had a talk to him. The great man realised at once that his new acquaintance had a distinguished and wide-ranging mind, and he invited the lad to visit him at his house in Tredrea. There, he said, young Davy would find a well-furnished scientific library of which he would be welcome to make use. Later, Giddy was to bring his young 'discovery' to the notice of a Doctor Edwards, who lived at the Copper House, near the Port of Hayle, and who was at that time Lecturer in Chemistry in the Medical School of St Bartholomew's Hospital in London. Doctor Edwards was as impressed by the young Humphry as Davies Giddy had been, and he suggested that the young man might like to make use of the apparatus in his own laboratory. As he got to know young Davy better, Doctor Edwards was able to indicate to him several invaluable fields of research.

Then, to Penzance, came some other notable men. First of these was Gregory Watt, son of James Watt the 'Father of the Steam Engine'. Young Gregory had been told that he ought to stay at Penzance for the sake of his health. He moved into lodgings in the home of Humphry Davy's widowed mother, and the two young men quickly became close friends. Humphry Davy was able to give Gregory Watt some valuable instruction in chemistry, and Watt was able to reciprocate with much information he had gathered from his father and his father's erudite friends.

Next came two learned geologists – a Doctor Thomas Beddoes and a Professor Hailstone. These two men were engaged at the time in a serious controversy over the subject in which they specialised, one preferring the 'Plutonian' and the other the 'Neptunist' hypothesis. In an attempt to settle the argument, they had decided to visit and to examine the Cornish coast, and they had made arrangements to be accompanied, while they were there, by Davies Giddy.

Doctor Beddoes, a Bristol physician with an enquiring mind, had foreseen a great future for 'pneumatic medicine' – a therapy in which 'factitious airs', or specially adapted gases, would be administered to a patient for the sufferer's benefit. In the early 1790s he had been experimenting with the effects of various gases on humans and animals. Hearing of Beddoes' experiments, other doctors had started to waft vapours, with alembics and bellows, over patients suffering from such varied troubles as asthma, dropsy, opium addiction and insanity. The Duchess of Devonshire had been among the influential visitors to Beddoes' laboratory. James Watt had become interested in the possibilities of 'pneumatic medicine', and he had been joined by Josiah Wedgwood, who had subscribed £1000 to advance the cause.

With all this distinguished support, Doctor Beddoes had recently been able to establish at Bristol a 'Pneumatic Institution' at which, he intended, there should be investigated fully the possible medical uses of artificially produced airs and gases. When the Doctor told Davies Giddy that he was looking for an assistant who would supervise the work being done at his Pneumatic Institution, Giddy had no hesitation in recommending for the post his young protégé Humphry Davy. Mrs Davy and John Borlase seem to have thought the idea a good one. John Tonkin violently opposed it and actually went as far as altering his will when he found that Davy insisted on joining Doctor Beddoes. On 2 October 1798, Davy took up his new post at Bristol.

Although Davy did not wish to give up altogether the profession of medicine – he still intended to study and graduate at Edinburgh – he soon found that his considerable energies were almost completely absorbed by the researches being carried out at the Pneumatic Institution. He ran, in the course of them, considerable risks. When he breathed in nitrous oxide, for instance, he found that the gas united with the common air in his mouth and formed nitrous acid, which severely injured his mucous membranes. When he tried inhaling carburetted hydrogen gas he 'seemed sinking into annihilation'. On being removed into the fresh air, he was heard to murmur faintly 'I do not think that I shall die',[1] but some hours passed before the painful symptoms disappeared.

Six months after he arrived at Bristol, Davy wrote to Davies Giddy to say 'I made a discovery yesterday which proves how necessary it is to repeat experiments. The gaseous oxide of azote (the laughing gas) is perfectly respirable when pure'.[2] He went on to tell Giddy that he had breathed sixteen quarts of it for nearly seven minutes, and that it had 'absolutely intoxicated'[3] him.

Doctor Beddoes, reporting in 1799 on the progress of the work of the Institution, expressed his great satisfaction with Humphry Davy's discovery of the properties of nitrous oxide, or laughing gas. When administered to Mrs Beddoes, the gas had produced 'pretty uniform pleasurable sens-ations',[4] with a propensity to muscular exertion. She had frequently 'seemed to ascend like a balloon'.[5] A patient named Tobin had experienced 'sometimes sublime emotions with tranquil gestures, sometimes violent muscular action, with sensations indescribably exquisite; no subsequent debility – no exhaustion'.[6] And the Revd Rochemont Barbauld had been 'exhilarated and compelled to laugh not by any ludicrous idea but by an impulse unconnected with thought and similar to that which is felt by children full of health and spirits'.[7]

Testimonials had been received, too, from a number of celebrities who had been persuaded to sniff the newly publicised gas. Samuel Taylor Coleridge had felt a sudden diffused warmth, a thrilling in the cheeks, arms and hands and a propensity to laugh. Robert Southey had reported some initial dizziness, followed by 'a peculiar thrilling in the extremities, a sensation perfectly new and delightful',[8] which was afterwards described as 'a new pleasure for which language has no name'.[9] Influenced, probably, by Dr. Beddoes, Davy published his *Researches, Chemical and Philosophical, chiefly concerning Nitrous Oxide and its Respiration* – a step which he was afterwards to regret, calling his immature hypotheses 'the dreams of misemployed genius which the light of experiment and observation has never conducted to truth'.

Though Dr Beddoes had such faith in nitrous oxide, believing that the gas might 'exalt the bodily and mental powers, enabling man to rule over the causes of pain and delight',[10] he was unable to prove that it had any curative powers, even when administered to such probable beneficiaries as the deaf, the hysterical and the paralysed. More, it had to be used with the greatest caution. There was an alarming incident when a highly-strung woman patient, who had inhaled an unsuitable mixture, had to be rushed into his home for emergency treatment. The Pneumatic Institution failed in 1801, unregretted by those residents of Bristol who had always suspected that it had been poisoning the surrounding air. 'Pneumatic medicine' did not disappear completely, though, for compression chambers, with and without medicated vapours, were included in the equipment of several well-patronised Victorian spas.

Although Davy did not remain satisfied for long with his *Researches, Chemical and Philosophical,* the work attracted a great deal of attention in scientific circles, and in July 1801 the young man was invited to join the Royal Institution in Albemarle Street, London, as an assistant lecturer in chemistry and as director of the Institution's chemical laboratories. Davy's lectures soon became popular and attracted many people from the higher ranks of London society. After the concluding lecture in a course that he called 'Pneumatic Chemistry' he administered nitrous oxide to several gentlemen present, who promptly rolled around, causing a minor sensation.

It seems remarkable now that the real significance of Humphry Davy's early work in the field of 'pneumatic chemistry' should not have been properly appreciated in medical circles for approximately forty years. As early as 1799, Davy had written, of nitrous oxide, that it 'seemed capable of destroying pain and might probably be used with advantage in surgical operations', but laughing gas continued to be used, even after that, as if it were merely an amusing toy. Demonstrations were given with it at fairgrounds and various houses of entertainment, causing much hilarity. Then, in 1815, Michael Faraday, Davy's assistant, noted that ether could be used to produce the same kind of intoxicating effect as nitrous oxide, and within a few years 'ether frolics' had become as popular with the jovially-minded as the 'laughing gas side shows' had been. One of the few men working in the first decades of the nineteenth century who appear to have treated Humphry Davy's Bristol researches with real respect was a Doctor Henry Hickman of Ludlow, in Shropshire. He published, in 1824, the results of some experiments he had been making with animals, claiming that unconsciousness and insensibility to pain could be produced if carbon dioxide gas were inhaled. This, Doctor Hickman suggested, might prove useful in surgery. No one would take Doctor Hickman's ideas seriously, however, and he was generally regarded as a crank and a bore. He died, it was said 'of a broken heart'[11] – at the early age of twenty-nine.

In a public garden at Boston, Massachusetts, there is a monument intended to remind passers-by of 'the discovery that the inhaling of ether causes insensibility to pain'. The name of the person who made that historic discovery is not to be seen on the monument, however, because no one knows for certain who really deserves the honour. It is generally conceded, though, that the great innovator was an American, and many medical historians believe that the credit should go to Crawford Williamson Long, before anyone else.

Long – a country practitioner of Jefferson, Georgia – was twenty-seven years old in 1842. He had been born, coincidentally, in the year in which Michael Faraday, on the other side of the Atlantic, had recorded for the first time the intoxicating powers of ether. Invited to take part in the fashionable 'ether frolics', Long had noticed that people who suffered bruises or other minor injuries while they were under the influence of the sweet-smelling gas did not appear to feel any pain. When he was required to excise a tumour from the neck of a boy called James Venable, Long decided that the boy should first inhale ether. The operation was painless and successful, and Long is believed to have used ether, after that, in other cases. Seven years elapsed, though, before Long, who was not fame-hungry, drew the attention of the medical world to his discovery. In the meantime some other pioneers had been at work, and they were a little more conscious than Long of the uses of publicity. In 1844, for instance, a man named Gardner Colton who gave lectures on chemical subjects paid a visit to the town of Hartford in Connecticut. Among the demonstrations Colton gave on this occasion was one which showed his audience the strange and amusing effects that could be produced if a human being were persuaded to inhale nitrous oxide gas. In the audience there happened to be a local dentist named Horace Wells who (like Crawford Long) had been born in 1815. As he watched the demonstration, Wells noticed that the 'victim' to whom the gas had been administered injured his leg in his excitement but appeared to feel no pain. On the following day, Wells asked Colton if he would kindly administer nitrous oxide to him so that a friend and colleague of his – a Doctor Riggs – could extract painlessly one of his molar teeth. Colton agreed to carry out the experiment, Doctor Riggs pulled out the offending tooth, and as Wells came back to consciousness he is said to have exclaimed, breathlessly, 'A new era in tooth pulling!'[12]

The start of the 'new era' was to be a little delayed, however, for after making a further trial of nitrous oxide gas in his dental practice and finding that it quite came up to his expectations, Wells ventured to give a public demonstration of the momentous new technique. On this occasion, unfortunately for Wells, things went wrong, and he was thoroughly discredited. The disappointment he suffered appears to have unbalanced him to some degree, for before long he abandoned dentistry altogether and took up picture dealing. Four years after he had collaborated with Gardner Colton and Doctor Riggs in the historic experiment at Hartford, Horace Wells committed suicide.[13]

The initiative, meanwhile, had passed to Wells's partner William Thomas Morton (born in 1819). Wells's enthusiasm for the new technique of 'painless dental extraction' undoubtedly influenced Morton in his subsequent career, for shortly after the two men, as a result of Wells's public discomfiture, had dissolved their partnership, Morton moved to Boston, where he went on quietly experimenting with nitrous oxide. As Wells had so unhappily discovered, Morton found, too, that nitrous oxide could have some entirely unpredictable side-effects, and he sought for some drug that would suppress pain as effectively as nitrous oxide but which would be considerably less capricious. 'Why don't you try ether?' suggested a Doctor Charles Jackson who, like Crawford Long, had been at one or more of the recently fashionable 'frolics'. Morton then tried ether on himself and on a dental patient named Eben Frost. It worked, and worked well, and Morton appears to have been entirely satisfied. Next, Morton decided to try a more or less public demonstration of his new discovery – probably he would want to be known professionally as a successful innovator. So he persuaded one of the Boston surgeons, named John Collins Warren, to allow him to give a demonstration of his methods before a number of medical men. This classic operation took place at the Massachusetts General Hospital on 16 October 1846, and it involved Warren making an incision in the neck of a young man called Gilbert Abbott. As the operation was successfully and painlessly completed, Warren is said to have pronounced, with pride, 'Gentlemen! This is no humbug!'[14]

But if there was no humbug about the use of the pain-killing ether, there were elements in the character of William Thomas Morton which were not entirely straightforward. Before him, Morton saw, were many years of successful pain-killing, during which he would be able to acquire a considerable fortune. To be fair to Morton he was not, properly speaking, a medical man, and therefore he would probably see no ethical reason for making his great discovery generally available, without charge, for the benefit of suffering humanity. So he tried to keep secret the identity of the drug he had been recommending, by adding colour to it and by disguising, as well as he could, its pungent odour. Aided and abetted by Charles Jackson, he even tried to patent ether, bestowing on it the evocative and unscientific name 'Letheon'. But Morton's subterfuges were soon exposed by some keen watchdog in the medical profession and the real nature and value of 'Letheon' became universally known.

There followed some lengthy and heated arguments about the claims that could properly be made for the proud title of Discoverer of Anaesthetics. Oliver Wendell Holmes proposed this name for the new advancement in medical science and it has remained in use ever since. The person who was awarded the title would be worthy of the gratitude of all mankind, and he would have to be financially rewarded, too. So the members of the United States Congress, remembering that the members of the British government had voted, earlier in the century, that sums totalling £30,000 should be presented to Edward Jenner after his discovery of vaccination, offered to give the sum of $100,000 to anyone who could prove that they, before anybody else, had developed and applied successfully an anaesthetic. Claims were made by

Long, Morton, Jackson and by members of the family of the deceased Horace Wells. The controversies that followed went on, intermittently, for years, but no such award was ever made and the issue has still not been finally resolved.

News of the great contribution made to the sum of human happiness by the small band of American innovators quickly reached the other continents, and soon there were a number of medical men in Europe who were eager to apply to their patients' advantage the information they had received from the United States. The first British 'anaesthetist' – using the word, here, to mean someone who devotes the greatest part of his professional time to the administration of anaesthetics – was a Doctor John Snow (born 1813) who, hearing from America of the historic experiments that had been made with ether, carried out, in an attempt to find some completely reliable method of administering the vapours, a number of careful experiments of his own. When he was satisfied that he had developed a thoroughly practical technique by these researches, Doctor Snow sought and was granted permission to demonstrate, in the room at St George's Hospital, London, that was reserved for dental out-patients, the results of his labours. The demonstration went off so well that from that time on and until his own health gave way almost all the 'ether practice' of London was left securely in Doctor Snow's competent hands.

There is no doubt about the time or place of the first major operation to be performed in Britain with the patient entirely under the influence of a general anaesthetic. The day was 21 December 1846; the place, the Hospital of University College in Gower Street, London. The hospital stood, and stands, only a few yards from the ground on which Robert Trevithick had demonstrated, earlier in the century, the first passenger-drawing steam locomotive.

The operation was performed on a butler named Frederick Churchill who was aged thirty-six, and it involved the amputation of one of Churchill's legs through the thigh. As such amputations had only been undertaken, in the days before anaesthetics were available, in dire emergencies when the use of the knife gave almost the only hope, and that a very slender one, of saving the patient's life, there can hardly have been much optimism engendered by the decision to operate. The anaesthetic was administered by one of the hospital's doctors, a Peter Squire. The surgeon was the tall and powerful Robert Liston.

Liston had been born in 1794 in the manse at Ecclesmachan, Linlithgowshire, where his father was the minister of the parish. After some medical training, Robert had been made a 'surgeon's clerk' at the Royal Infirmary of Edinburgh. He had travelled to London in 1816, and had attended John Abernethy's lectures at St Bartholomew's Hospital. From 1818 to 1828, Liston had worked once more in Edinburgh. There were few surgeons of any consequence to be found, in those days, outside the great towns, and he was made operating surgeon at the Royal Infirmary there in the latter year. In 1833, Liston suffered a grievous disappointment when the Chair of Clinical Surgery at Edinburgh became vacant, and he failed to be appointed to it, his rival and former colleague James Syme (born 1799) being preferred by the authorities. As soon as a suitable opportunity offered, Liston moved south again, and shortly afterwards was offered the Chair of Clinical Surgery in the University of London.

Liston was noted in medical and surgical circles for his satirical tongue and his uncertain temper. He was famous, too, for his nerves of steel. There was no place, in the agonising scenes that had to be enacted in a pre-anaesthetics operating theatre, for a surgeon who hesitated, or whose judgement was affected by the emotions of pity or remorse. He was also renowned for the speed and dexterity with which he could perform his operations. This, when the patient was suffering indescribable torments, and when time was of the essence, took precedence over all other requirements. It was said of Liston that when he performed an amputation the gleam of his knife was followed so instantaneously by the sound of sawing as to make the two actions appear almost simultaneous. For the first time ever, on that dark December day in the operating theatre by Gower Street, London, Robert Liston was able to take his time. After he had finished the operation, he is said to have observed coolly to those who had been watching him that 'this Yankee dodge beats Mesmerism hollow'.[15]

When, in 1846, news reached Scotland of the operations that had been performed in America with the aid of ether, the potential importance of the new techniques was appreciated at once by James Young Simpson – another son of Linlithgowshire, who, at the age of twenty-eight, had been appointed Professor of Midwifery at Edinburgh University. Simpson had already witnessed, in his large and constantly expanding practice, a distressing amount of human misery. 'It is a glorious thought, I can think of naught else',[16] he wrote of the new vista of painless childbirth that had suddenly opened up before him. As quickly as he could, he arranged the first trials of ether ever to be made in the field of midwifery. These trials were not unsuccessful, but Professor Simpson was soon to decide that a more efficient and a more readily portable general anaesthetic than ether should be sought for. He was still looking urgently for an 'improved' anaesthetic when David Waldie, a Liverpool chemist, suggested to him that he might like to try chloroform.

Chloroform had been discovered by a New York chemist named Guthrie some fifteen years before. (Guthrie described his 'new mode of preparing a spirituous solution of chloric ether' in the *American Journal of Science and Arts*, published in 1831–2 at New Haven). It had also been discovered in France, at approximately the same time, by a M. Soubeiran, who knew nothing of Guthrie's researches, and who described his own findings in *Les Annales de Chimie, Volume XLVIII*, published in 1831. In Germany, the great chemist J. von Liebig published his own notes on the subject during 1832. In 1835 it had been prepared, described, and first given the name 'chloroform' by a M. Jean-Baptiste Dumas, of

Paris. None of these chemists had supposed that chloroform would be of any great practical use, and up to that time it had, in fact, only been administered internally. James Simpson decided to follow up David Waldie's suggestion, however, and he resolved to try inhaling its fumes.

During the evening of 4 November 1847, then, James Simpson and his assistants Doctors George Keith and Duncan assembled for the purpose of testing the pain-killing powers of chloroform. A supply of the proposed anaesthetic had been prepared for them by Messrs. Duncan, Flockhart and Company, of Edinburgh. The trial was only too successful – the new drug rapidly took effect and the three men passed out simultaneously, almost as if they had been shot. As Simpson recovered consciousness and saw his colleagues still lying helpless under the table at which they had been sitting he said to himself, he was to recall later: 'This is far stronger than ether'.[17]

On 10 November 1847 – less than a week after his bold experiment – Simpson gave *An Account of a New Anaesthetic Agent* to the Edinburgh Medico-Chirurgical Society. Five days later, at the Royal Edinburgh Infirmary, he administered chloroform to a boy from the Highlands who could speak only Gaelic. The boy, suffering from osteomyelitis, was to have part of a radius bone removed by Simpson's colleague Professor James Miller. The operation was carried out successfully. It looked, then, as though Simpson's courageous innovation had been fully justified, but before the use of chloroform could be more widely accepted he had to face many bitter attacks from prejudiced members of the lay public who claimed that the new drug was dangerous to health and that the use of it was 'going against religion'. It was some time before the chorus of denunciation died down.

During the next fifty years, chloroform was the anaesthetic chosen by most of the surgeons in Britain and in many other parts of the world, and much of the credit for its almost universal acceptance can be given to Doctor John Snow.

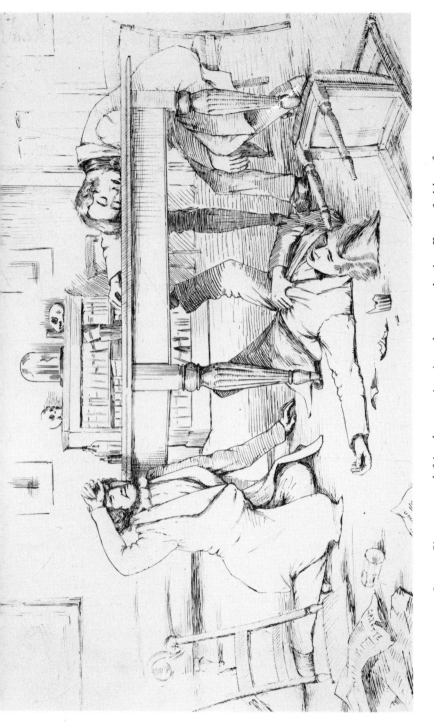

James Simpson and friends experiencing the anaesthetic effect of chloroform

Although he was acknowledged to be the country's leading expert in the use of ether, Snow was too wise and too open-minded to ignore any other possible anaesthetics that might be made available, and when he heard about James Simpson's adventures with chloroform he carried out some extensive researches in a determined effort to find the best way in which the new drug might be used. He described these researches in his book *On Chloroform and other Anaesthetics* which was published in 1858. On two occasions – when Prince Leopold was born in 1853, and again when Princess Beatrice was born in 1857 – Snow administered chloroform to Her Majesty Queen Victoria.

The risks that were cheerfully and courageously taken by so many of the great medical and surgical pioneers of the nineteenth century can hardly be underestimated by anyone who thinks carefully about the unprecedented steps into the unknown that were taken by such men as James Simpson and his assistants. In some cases, of course, such experiments were bound to end in tragedy. One of the most notable victims of the 'experiment on oneself' urge was Doctor Joseph Toynbee.

Joseph Toynbee – born, like those other researchers in the field of anaesthetics, in the year 1815 – was a native of Lincolnshire, where his father was a well-to-do farmer. After spending some years at King's Lynn Grammar School, Joseph was apprenticed, at the age of eighteen, to a William Wade, who worked at the Westminster General Dispensary which was situated in Gerrard Street, near Leicester Square. He studied anatomy at the nearby Little Windmill Street School, and then attended St George's Hospital and the University College Hospital, being admitted to membership of the College of Surgeons in 1838.

All through the years he spent as a student in London, Joseph Toynbee was especially interested in diseases of the ear, which, he felt, had been largely neglected by members of the medical and surgical professions – neglected, in fact, to such an extent that the study of otology was in danger of passing entirely into the hands of 'quack' doctors. Publicly, he vowed to do what he could to rescue aural pathology from the charlatans' monopolistic attentions, and to convert it, as well as he could, into a more exact science.

In pursuit of his aims, Toynbee made more than two thousand dissections of human ears, most of the ears being taken after death from patients whose weaknesses and ailments Toynbee had been studying prior to their demise. A large number of his most important researches were described in his book *Diseases of the Ear* which ranks, still, as a medical classic. As early as 1836 he was writing authoritative letters about diseases of the ear to the Lancet, and when St Mary's Hospital, London, was established in 1851 – it was the first general hospital, anywhere, to have beds set aside specially for patients suffering from diseases of the ear – he was almost automatically elected to be its aural surgeon and to be the lecturer, in its medical school, on this subject: posts that he held with the greatest distinction until 1864.

In 1886, Toynbee was acting as aural surgeon to the Ea:'swood Asylum for Idiots and as consulting aural surgeon to the Asylum for the Deaf and Dumb, as well as holding a number of other posts, some of them being concerned, chiefly, with philanthropic work. He was becoming increasingly preoccupied too, with the intense suffering that many of his patients had to undergo when they were unfortunate enough to be stricken with certain inflammatory conditions of the middle ear. Could he, he wondered, by research and experiment, find a way of lessening that suffering?

The answer – he decided – might have something to do with the inhalation of chloroform. If chloroform were inhaled, so that the ear might subsequently be inflated . . . would that have a positive, pain-relieving effect?

With great courage, Joseph Toynbee decided to subject himself to the crucial test. He was found dead, later, in his consulting room, with his research notes and all the necessary apparatus by his side. The fame of his second son Arnold, who appears to have inherited Joseph's philanthropic ideals, is perpetuated now by the benevolent community 'Toynbee Hall' in the East End of London.

# 6

# *Antiseptics*

From the beginning of time until the middle of the
nineteenth century, surgery of any kind was liable and even
likely to be followed by infection, and infection was liable,
and even likely, to prove fatal.

The idea that infection might be caused by the unseen
entry into the body of tiny, invisible organisms had been
kicked around for at least two thousand years. It was given
publicity by the Roman encyclopaedist Varro a hundred
years before the birth of Christ. It was repeated by Fracas-
toro and by Athanasius Kircher and Pierre Borel in the
sixteenth and seventeenth centuries. In 1684, Francesco Redi
wrote a remarkable work which he called *Observations on
Living Animals which are to be found inside Other Living Animals.*
In this, he attempted to refute the theory of spontaneous
generation. Everything must have a parent, he asserted. Only
life can produce life.

Then, in 1720, Richard Mead, a London physician who
had graduated at the University of Padua, published his *Short
Discourse Concerning Pestilential Contagion and the Methods to be
used to Prevent it.* In this book, Doctor Mead stated positively
that the poor were 'most obnoxious to contagious diseases'
because they were overcrowded and lacked cleanliness. Mead

57

gave specific instructions, too, for keeping in quarantine those who were suffering from infectious diseases; for the evacuation of towns affected by the plague; for the cleansing or destruction of houses that had harboured people who had been suffering from the more obnoxious diseases; and for the prohibition of public assemblies when epidemics were rife. The advice Mead gave would be commended by any responsible municipal officer today.

Not much more headway than that had been made by the start of the nineteenth century. Relatively few people who were operated on in the overcrowded hospitals actually survived the dreaded post-surgical period, when the flesh that had been cut would start, with tragic inevitability, to suppurate. With the dice loaded so heavily against them, the surgeons of those days were forced to limit their activities to the performance of emergency operations, such as the amputation of limbs or parts of limbs that were dangerously damaged, the removal of stones, and minor repairs to the outer surfaces of the body. Major surgical work on the cavities of the chest or the abdomen was made virtually impossible by the undisputed risk of sepsis.

Some, at least, of the surgeons who were working in the hospitals at the beginning of the nineteenth century suspected that there might be some connection between dirt and sepsis. A few were even bold enough to speak out against the overcrowded conditions in which surgical patients were kept. They protested, too, against the number of patients with 'dirty' or suppurating wounds who might be expected to share a single ward. The majority of the surgeons went on unwittingly infecting their patients, however, every time they used a knife. They wore their oldest frock coats in the operating theatre – coats that were stiffly encrusted with the dried blood and pus of previous patients. From the buttonholes of these coats they would hang, until these were needed, the pieces of whipcord that they used for tying the arteries of their patients. The probes with which they examined the wounds of their patients were never sterilized and might not even be washed. It is surprising that any patients at all managed to survive operations carried out under these appalling conditions.

Faced with the apparently insuperable problems of post-operative sepsis, most surgeons of the time tended to favour some technique by which, they optimistically believed, the ravages of suppuration might be limited. Some, who had noticed that once a healthy scab had formed on a wound, that wound would be more likely to progress satisfactorily, preferred to leave all wounds uncovered, to encourage encrustation. Others, who believed that sepsis might be caused by a kind of poison carried in the air, used to seal off wounds with air-tight dressings, such as those made with gold-beaters' skin. If a wound were already infected, this technique would seal in the infective organisms and would usually prove fatal. One of the few moderately successful techniques was evolved by the prominent Edinburgh surgeon James Syme (1799–1870), who used to leave the long ends of ligatures hanging out, so that the infective matter in the wounds of his patients would drain out into their dressings. Such expedients were, however, little more than desperate attempts to stem an unstoppable tide.

One notable and relevant discovery – predating by several years the discovery of the part played by bacteria in the transmission of disease – was made by Doctor John Snow, who has already been discussed in connection with the use of anaesthetics.

Snow, apprenticed to a surgeon at Newcastle-on-Tyne, had served as an unqualified assistant during the great cholera epidemic of 1831–2, and he had had an excellent opportunity to study at first hand the agonizing effects of the disease, or, as we know now, of this group of diseases. Cholera patients seen by Snow would be suffering from acute diarrhoea accompanied, usually, by vomiting. As they became increasingly dehydrated, they would be liable to be tormented by severe muscular cramps and their thirst would be intense. In the later stages of the disease, many of the patients would become comatose, and in the worst cases would die of shock.

In October 1836, Snow became a student at the Hunterian School in Great Windmill Street, and there he learned the value of a truly scientific approach in any important investigation. By compiling a list of the most serious outbreaks of cholera, and by studying the dates and situations of those outbreaks, he found that cholera appeared to have moved slowly westward from India, taking several centuries to reach Paris and London, where the disease had become a serious threat to public health by 1849. With rare scientific insight, Snow then evolved the theory that cholera is spread through the agency of a contaminated water supply.

It was the dreadful cholera epidemic of 1854 that gave Snow his first real chance to show that the disease might be communicated by the crude sanitary arrangements prevailing at the time. There was, he found, in Golden Square a public well known as the Broad Street Pump, and he managed to establish that this well was being contaminated through leakage from a nearby sewer. We know for certain, now, that Snow was right – the bacteria *Vibrio Cholerae*, sometimes called, because of its curved shape, '*Vibrio Comma*', enters the body through the mouth, usually in contaminated water or food. From there, it travels to the mucous membranes that line the lumen of the small intestine – a refinement that Snow could not possibly have known. For confirmation about bacterial infection, the world had to await the researches of Joseph Lister and Louis Pasteur.

Joseph Lister was born at Upton Park, in the parish of West Ham, a little to the east of the City of London, on 5 April 1827. His parents were Quakers, and wealthy. His father – Joseph Jackson Lister – devoted most of the time when he was not actively engaged in the family's wine business to the study of physics and microscopy. In 1832, Joseph Jackson was elected to a Fellowship of the Royal Society, principally because he had written a paper that dealt with the properties of an 'achromatic' microscope lens: a lens which would protect the viewer from the dazzling iridescence caused by strong white light that had baffled earlier researchers.

When Joseph Lister the younger left the nursery, both his parents actively encouraged him to widen his interests, his father directing him particularly towards natural history and the uses of the microscope. The Quaker schools to which he was sent were unusual for the time, in that they laid particular emphasis on the importance of science, and virtually ignored the study of the classics. Before Joseph Lister had reached the age of sixteen, he had developed a very real interest in comparative anatomy, and had already set his heart on becoming a surgeon.

After taking an arts course at University College, London, Lister enrolled, in October 1848, in the Faculty of Medical Science. While he was a student, he heard about the first surgical operation to be carried out in Britain with the aid of a general anaesthetic. No mention of this historic operation is to be found in Lister's letters, though it certainly had a profound influence on his future career.

Lister, it is known, was a brilliant student. He graduated with honours as a Bachelor of Medicine in 1852, and in the same year was made a Fellow of the Royal College of Surgeons and appointed House Surgeon at University College Hospital. He was particularly interested in physiology which, he wrote, 'is even more important to the surgeon than it is to the physician'. The results of his researches were sufficiently informative to merit publication in the *Quarterly Journal of Microscopical Science*.

In the following year, Lister made a journey to Scotland at the suggestion of his Professor of Physiology, William Sharpey, who recognized the potentialities of this exceptional young man and believed that he would benefit by studying briefly in Edinburgh under James Syme, who was then regarded as the foremost surgeon in Britain and – in the opinion of many authorities – in Europe too. Armed with a letter of introduction from Professor Sharpey to Professor Syme, Lister left London intending to spend a month in the

Scottish capital. He was to stay for much longer than that.

Attracted, probably, by Lister's independence of mind, Syme took to the young man from London and, before the end of the month, urged him not to return to England. In the year after Lister's arrival in Edinburgh, Syme made him his house surgeon. Lister was in charge of twelve dressers who referred to him, not disrespectfully, as 'The Chief', a nickname that he was to keep for the rest of his life. 'I must not expect to be a Liston or a Syme', he wrote to his father. 'Still, I shall get on. Certain it is that I love surgery more and more, and . . . I am honest and a lover of truth, which is as important as anything . . .'[1]

Backed enthusiastically by Syme, Lister did indeed 'get on'. When R.J. Mackenzie – a clever young Edinburgh surgeon – died of cholera while he was serving in the Crimea,[2] Lister was chosen to succeed him as Assistant Surgeon to the Edinburgh Royal Infirmary and as Lecturer in Surgery in the Extra-Mural School. Syme gave Lister every encouragement, too, when the young man paid court to his eldest daughter Agnes. The pair were married on 23 April 1856, after which Lister, who was an upright man, felt morally obliged to sever his links with the Quaker community, joining instead the Scottish Episcopal Church, to which his wife and her family belonged.

For thirty-nine years after that, Lister's wife was also his principal assistant. Not having to cope with some of the Victorian housewife's more demanding chores – for the couple remained childless – Mrs Lister acted as her husband's secretary, writing notes and letters to his dictation for many hours without taking a rest. She looked after his surgical instruments, too, and helped him with his experiments. And she tried to make a punctual man of him, but this proved difficult, for Lister would often become so totally absorbed in his work that he would be quite unaware of his next appointment.

In spite of his growing reputation in Edinburgh's surgical circles, Lister was not at this stage of his career very successful at attracting private clients. Mrs Lister used to speak of 'Poor Joseph and his one patient'.[3] He was therefore able to spend a considerable proportion of his time on researches into such subjects as the part that the blood vessels play in the first stages of inflammation and the mechanism of the coagulation of the blood. All these researches depended on the use of the microscope and were directly connected with the healing of wounds.

In 1859, the Regius Professorship of Surgery at Glasgow became vacant, and Lister decided to apply for this important post, which was in the gift of the Government, the Home Secretary being in this respect its most influential member. The post would carry with it a satisfactory salary, Lister saw, and it would be a useful stepping stone to any surgical professorship that might fall vacant, either in Edinburgh or, preferably, London. He realised, too, that he would be free, in Glasgow, from his celebrated father-in-law's constant supervision, much as he had appreciated this in his early days at Edinburgh. By this time, he was more interested in developing his own ideas.

In spite of some interference by the two Glasgow M.P.s, Lister was chosen, in preference to the six other candidates. The official notification from the Home Secretary's Private Secretary reached him on 28 January 1860. Proudly, he wrote to his father on the following day: 'It made us almost intoxicated with gladness, doubled or trebled, I doubt not, by the long period of suspense which had preceded it. Indeed I never remember having experienced before such great and unmixed satisfaction at any intelligence'.[4]

His new post, and the position of Surgeon to the Glasgow Royal Infirmary to which he was appointed in August 1861, offered Lister plenty of scope for research. The wards in the new surgical block at the Infirmary – wards of which he was officially in charge – were noteworthy. The Infirmary Managers had put up these wards in the hope that the dreaded 'hospital diseases', which included the disease now known as 'post-operative sepsis', would be greatly decreased by their enterprise. Their hopes proved vain, however, for the wards had been built on the site of an old burial ground that was filled with coffins containing the rotting bodies of victims of the great cholera epidemic of 1849, and were said to be some of the most unhealthy in the kingdom. Lister found that in his male accident ward, during the years 1861 to 1865, a depressingly high percentage of his amputation cases died from sepsis.

Lister knew at the time that most of the current theories about post-operative sepsis were incorrect – the belief, for instance, that it was caused by 'miasma' or direct infection by bad air was particularly misleading – but he also had some sound thinking and observation on which to base the next extensions of his work. He knew, for example, that Oliver Wendell Holmes, the great American physician, poet, and humorist, who had been made Professor of Anatomy and Physiology at Harvard in 1847, had, four years before that, directed the attention of the whole of the American medical profession to the contagious quality of puerperal fever, and had suggested, with characteristic incisiveness, that doctors might themselves be the most active carriers of disease. Lister knew, too, that the dreaded 'hospital diseases' attacked only those patients who had broken skins. A simple fracture where the skin was intact would usually mend quite readily, whereas a compound fracture with its open wound would as often as not lead to suppuration. Quite shortly after he arrived in Glasgow, Lister was pointing this out to his students. Anyone, he said, who could explain this difference and enable open wounds to behave like closed wounds would be among the greatest benefactors of the age. And, he added, the evils of 'hospitalism' – gangrene, erysipelas and pyaemia – were encountered much more frequently in hospitals than in private houses. In the largest hospitals, he would add, these evils flourished most outrageously of all. Why, he would ask, was that?

It was Thomas Anderson, Professor of Chemistry in Glasgow, who first drew Lister's attention to the great work that was being done on the Continent by the French chemist Louis Pasteur. Lister should study some papers on fermentation that Pasteur had recently published, suggested Anderson. They could contain material relevant to the study of the putrefaction of flesh which, at that time, was engaging so much of Lister's attention. Lister sent for the papers at once.

Louis Pasteur was born in 1822 at Dôle, a little town in the Jura. His father, a veteran of the Napoleonic Wars, earned his living as a tanner. Louis was educated at Artois and at the Royal College of Besançon where, in 1840, he was made 'Bachelier ès Lettres'. He became an assistant mathematics master in the College and, continuing to study, he was awarded in 1842 the 'Baccalaureat ès Sciences'. In 1843 he was admitted to the École Normale and there he started to attend the lectures given by J.B. Dumas at the Sorbonne. These roused his interest in chemistry and he decided to study the subject in earnest.

By 1852, Pasteur had been appointed Professor of Chemistry at Strasbourg. At this time, he was devoting much of his attention to isomeric compounds, making a classic investigation into the crystals of tartaric and para-tartaric acid that earned him, in 1856, the Rumford Medal of the Royal Society. Before that time, though, Pasteur had become intensely interested in the processes of fermentation and in the diseases of beer, milk, and wine.

In 1854, Pasteur was appointed Professor of Chemistry at the new Faculty of Sciences at Lille. At Lille, he was in a district where much alcohol was produced from grain and beet sugar, and he was able to carry out some intensive research into the causes of fermentation. On examining the yeasts of sound and 'sour' beer under a microscope, he saw that the globules of yeast in the sound beer were nearly spherical, while those in the unsound beer were elongated. He continued his researches until, in 1857, he was able to announce with complete conviction that fermentation is caused by minute organisms. If a fermentation fails, he asserted, the cause must be the absence of the necessary organisms or the failure of those organisms to grow. He demonstrated his point by adding to fresh milk organisms from buttermilk which quickly turned the fresh milk sour. He showed, too, that beer could be kept from turning sour if air and the spoiling organisms were rigorously excluded.

Next, Pasteur started a series of elaborate experiments which were intended to tell him more about the invisible organisms that interested him so keenly. Were they always present in the atmosphere? Were they spontaneously generated? After exposing unfermented liquids to filtered air and to the pure air of Alpine peaks, Pasteur was able to declare, with confidence, that the minute organisms that caused fermentation were not spontaneously generated. They were produced by similar organisms that were present, normally, in ordinary unfiltered air. The air of warm rooms and the polluted atmosphere of cities were particularly heavily stocked with these tiny self-multiplying organisms, Pasteur found.

It would have been surprising if all the more conservative scientists of the time had readily accepted Pasteur's revolutionary new ideas without demur. As it was, his announcements provoked fierce opposition. Among the most vocal of his opponents was the powerful Baron Von Liebig, who was widely regarded as being the most successful chemist of the day. Von Liebig studied Pasteur's propositions, but said that he preferred to believe that fermentation and putrefaction were processes which resembled some slow form of chemical combustion. Von Liebig's views were supported by many people connected with the study of chemistry, but as the Master resolutely refused to take even one single look into a microscope his views proved extremely difficult to defend.

As soon as Joseph Lister, in Scotland, heard that Louis Pasteur, in France, had shown that organic decomposition was not caused by bad air or by the spontaneous generation of germs but by living organisms carried through the air, usually on minute particles of dust, the Glasgow surgeon realised that the work being done by the great French scientist offered a straightforward solution to the dreadful enigmas over which he, Lister, had been puzzling for so long. His patients at the Royal Infirmary were suffering 'in a way that was sickening and often heart-rending, so as to make me feel it a questionable privilege to be connected with the institution'.[5] Could not his patients' agonies be caused by micro-organisms which found their way, unseen, to the surface of their wounds?

To find out if this theory would stand up, Lister realised that he would have to take a number of wounds and he would have to destroy any harmful micro-organisms that might be alive in them; then, he would have to prevent any further micro-organisms from reaching the wounds. If the wounds healed, after that, without suppurating, it would seem as though his reasoning were correct.

Pasteur had shown how harmful micro-organisms that happened to be in a liquid could be destroyed or rendered harmless by heat. He had shown, too, how harmful micro-organisms carried like pollen through the air might be removed from the air by a simple form of filtration. Lister preferred to use Pasteur's third method – a chemical method – of destroying the unwanted micro-organisms in, and approaching, the subjects of his studies. The Glasgow surgeon had come across a newly developed liquid called 'phenol' or 'carbolic acid', which had been prepared by a Manchester chemist named Calvert, and which had been used to disinfect and deodorise the sewage works at Carlisle. (It had been used as a disinfectant by a Parisian chemist named Jules Lemaire, too, though Lister was not aware of this at the time.) With carbolic acid, Lister guessed, the microscopic invaders might be easily and completely destroyed.

Lister made his initial experiments in March 1865, using, for the first test case, a patient who had a compound fracture of the leg. This was an ideal case for such a trial. The patient's condition could hardly become more dangerous, whatever damage might be accidentally done by a well-meaning doctor. Lister's experiments offered at least an outside chance of saving the limb.

The system of antisepsis Lister used in his early tests seems now so unsophisticated that it was, in itself, a source of possible danger. In applying directly to human tissues undiluted carbolic acid or various forms of putty or plaster that contained undiluted carbolic acid he was being more rigorous than he need have been. At first, he tried to protect his patients against the irritant action of the acid by the use of insulating materials, such as oiled silk and tinfoil. Later, however, he discovered that the application of weaker fluids that contained relatively small quantities of carbolic acid was just as effective, and did much less damage.

Besides applying carbolic acid directly to the wounds of his patients, Lister tried to ensure that anyone or anything that could touch or even approach the wounds – his instruments, the dressings, his own fingers and those of the dressers and nurses – should be treated with the antiseptic fluid. The extraordinary degree of success that Lister achieved, right from the start, with his antiseptic techniques was due to the thoroughness with which the new principles of surgery were applied. Two years after he carried out the first of his 'carbolic acid' operations, Lister was able to announce, in *The Lancet*, some startlingly successful results. He headed his historic article 'On a New Method of Treating Compound Fracture'. In it, he described eleven cases. Nine of his patients had survived and had become sound again in wind and limb. One had had to undergo an amputation. Only one out of the eleven had died. In the successful operations he had carried out by the new method, Lister claimed, his patients' blood had clotted satisfactorily, instead of becoming putrid. Their bodies, after that, had had a proper chance to recover.

A year later he wrote a further article, for the *British Medical Journal*, calling this 'On the Antiseptic System of Treatment in Surgery'. In this second article, Lister described his methods in some detail, and he let the world know how highly he valued carbolic acid as a material by means of which human lives might be saved.

It might, conceivably, have been better if Lister had not written about the virtues of carbolic acid in quite such eulogistic terms, for people were soon saying publicly, and incorrectly, that Lister had claimed to be the first person to use carbolic acid for the betterment of the human condition. This caused much bitterness among those who had been using carbolic acid for various useful purposes before Lister had selected it for his own urgent needs. Lister repeatedly disclaimed, after that, that he had set any very special store by carbolic acid. It was a chemical that had just happened to be conveniently available, he said, when he first started to use his 'antiseptic method'. Any other chemical would have done as well as long as it had been capable of destroying unwanted micro-organisms.

Encouraged by the success of his antiseptic method of surgery, Lister proceeded to carry out a number of other important experiments. From his Christmas holiday in 1868 until the end of his working life, for example, he was ceaselessly attempting, in the most painstaking way, to improve the range and quality of the ligatures available to the surgeon. Up to that time, most surgeons had used silk for tying blood-vessels and for similar purposes, but silk was not absorbed by the body or disposed of naturally in any other way, and ligatures made with it tended to cause irritation which, in turn, could lead to sepsis and other troubles. There was an urgent need, Lister saw, for some less permanent material that could be used in place of silk.

Lister's first really important discovery in this field was that catgut was absorbable, and a highly desirable substitute for silk. He confirmed catgut's advantages by tying with it the carotid artery of a living calf. One month later, when the calf was killed, Lister was pleased to find that the catgut had disappeared. In its place, there was a living ring of fibrous tissue. This discovery strengthened Lister's conviction that many notable benefits to humanity can only be expected if a reasonable number of experiments are carried out on living animals. Soon, Lister was showing his students how catgut ligatures could be made even safer if they were stored, until they were needed, in carbolised oil.

In 1869, James Syme was struck down with paralysis, from which he was to die in a few months. Lister was persuaded to return to Edinburgh to succeed his father-in-law in the Chair of Surgery there. The next few years were probably the happiest of Lister's life – he was becoming increasingly famous, and he was very popular with his students – but he had no chance to sit back to savour the fruits of his success: he was much too busy.

Soon after he arrived in Edinburgh, Lister managed to produce an 'antiseptic atmosphere' in which his operations could be carried out. He did this by means of a spray that sent out a fine mist of carbolic lotion into the air. The spray was worked, in the first place, by hand. Then a pump or 'donkey engine' was devised to vaporise and disseminate the dis-infectant. This, in its turn, was replaced by a larger steam engine which chugged away happily for more than twenty years, puffing out into the air round Lister's surgical patients the revolutionary and at that time almost invaluable dis-infectant vapours.

Soon after he arrived in Edinburgh, Lister managed to popularise the rubber drainage tube which had been first used by a French surgeon named Chassignac a few years before. One of the earliest of Lister's patients to have the benefit of this tube was Queen Victoria, who developed, during 1871, an abscess in the armpit. Lister went to Balmoral to open the royal abscess. Sir William Jenner, the Physician to the Royal Household, had also been required to attend. So Jenner was asked, diplomatically, to operate, by hand, the bellows of Lister's antiseptic spray. The operation was completely successful, and Lister earned Her Majesty's warm-hearted approval. He was to lose it, though, a few years later, when the Queen, who was a notable animal-lover, asked him to make a public statement condemning the 'awful' practice of

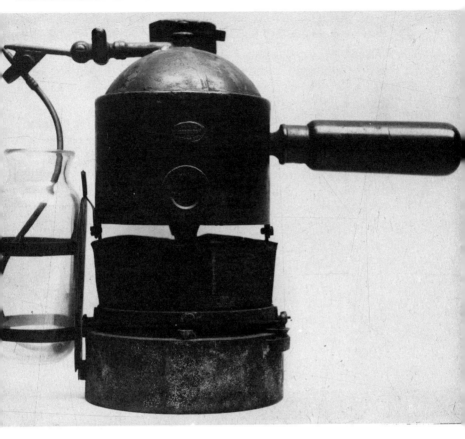

A Lister carbolic spray

vivisection, which was then being discussed by a Royal Commission.[6] Lister, remembering all too clearly the calf which had had to sacrifice its life in a recent good cause, tried, in a tactful reply, to explain to Her Majesty why he was in no position to do any such thing. The Queen was not amused, and Lister, in consequence, did not get until several more years had elapsed the baronetcy he so obviously deserved.

Lister's clinic at Edinburgh attracted, as was only to be expected, many distinguished – and curious – visitors from abroad, and there were others who sought advice and help from the great man through the post. Mathias Hieronymus Saxtorph (1822–1900), Professor of Clinical Surgery at Copenhagen, was one of the first men on the Continent to understand and embrace Lister's antiseptic principles. In a letter written to Lister in 1870 he reported that he had managed to banish pyaemia from his wards. Just Lucas-Championnière (1843–1913), who had trained under Lister at Glasgow, was the first person to advocate 'Listerism' in France. He published, in 1876, a short book entitled *Chirurgie Antiseptique*. Georg F.L. Stromeyer, who was a pioneer of orthopaedic surgery, was only one of Lister's many disciples in Germany, but he is particularly remembered because he was inspired to celebrate Lister's achievements in light verse:

Mankind looks grateful now on thee
    For what thou did'st in Surgery,
And Death must often go amiss,
    By smelling antiseptic bliss.

Theodore Billroth (1829–94), who taught and did much experimental surgery at Vienna, adopted Lister's methods at an early stage of his career, and so was able to carry out successfully, for the first time, such daring operations as the removal of stomach cancers and laryngectomies. From Vienna, Billroth's pupils carried Lister's teachings into many other parts of Europe. Lister himself was encouraged to travel. In 1875, he was invited to visit Germany and was given a rousing welcome. In the following year, he went to an international congress in Philadelphia, where he was just as enthusiastically received.

Then, in 1877, the year in which Lister celebrated his fiftieth birthday, Sir William Fergusson died, in London, leaving vacant the Chair of Clinical Surgery at the University's King's College. Lister heard the news with the greatest interest, for although his teachings on the importance of antiseptic techniques had been accepted, by that time, in almost every other part of the world, they had made remarkably little impact on the intensely conservative medical men of the English capital. This was not for want of trying on the part of Lister and his wife. Contemporary reports describe graphically the travels made by the industrious pair as they moved to, and between, a variety of medical meetings in the Metropolis, nursing carefully on their knees in cabs and railway carriages the famous flasks, filled with fermenting and boiled wine, with which they were attempting to demonstrate to unbelievers the truth of the relevant propositions of Louis Pasteur.[7] They were listened to, in London, with politeness, but with extraordinarily little enthusiasm.

When Lister was invited to fill the vacant Chair at King's College, London, he decided to accept. His students in Edinburgh were horrified, and seven hundred of them put their signatures to a petition that almost literally begged him to stay on in the Scottish capital. Lister, a man with a sense of mission, ignored their pleas.

The Listers moved to London, taking as their assistants two of the men – Watson Cheyne and John Stewart – who had been most useful to Lister in Scotland. Their reception was less than welcoming. The students, they found, were much less appreciative than the young men of Glasgow and Edinburgh. The nurses, disliking the extra and bothersome chores that were inseparable from the new-fangled antiseptic form of surgery, were openly antagonistic. Lister's professional associates were, in the main, scornful of him or just indifferent. Some of the more critical of them said openly that they were shocked when he operated on the knee joint to wire a fractured patella, but they were less caustic when Lister's apparent daring produced some most satisfactory results. Soon, even those who had scoffed the loudest were won over, and Lister's system was adopted as wholeheartedly in London as it had been in more readily receptive places.

During the 1880s, Lister decided to stop using his famous

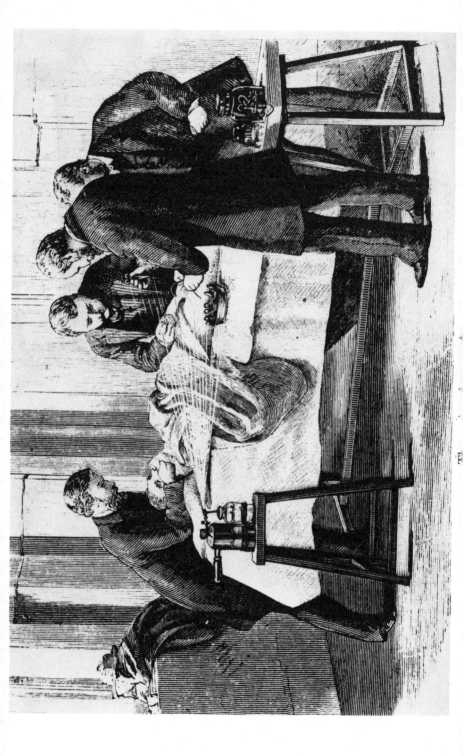

'antiseptic spray'. He had changed his ideas considerably since he had developed the original hand-operated diffuser, and by this time he was using gauzes impregnated with carbolic acid. Later, he was to use even more sophisticated methods than that. Before he had finished operating, he was relying on double cyanide gauze, which was charged with the cyanides of mercury and zinc, and was dyed a deep purple colour so that it could be instantly identified. By some, Lister's abandonment of his famous spray was taken as an indication that he had begun to lose faith in his antiseptic methods, but these people were soon shown that they were wrong.

While Lister was working away earnestly in London, Louis Pasteur, in France, was conducting a series of experiments that were to lead triumphantly to the further development of preventive inoculation. Edward Jenner had firmly established the science of immunology in the eighteenth century, but not much more progress had been made, except with respect to smallpox, since his day.

Pasteur's discoveries in this field started almost by chance. He had been investigating the disease known to poultry-keepers as 'chicken cholera', and the micro-organism which caused this trouble had already been isolated and identified. One evening, he inoculated a chicken with a culture made with the chicken cholera germs. By a chance that now seems almost miraculous, the culture was some six weeks old, and, to use a layman's term, might have been called a 'stale' one. The fowl became ill, but not seriously so, and then it recovered completely. Using the same bird and a fresh culture of virulent micro-organisms, Pasteur was fascinated to find that although the germs were highly dangerous to any uninoculated chicken, the treated bird appeared to have become resistant to the infection. The great Frenchman was quick to appreciate the historic importance of his discovery. The oxygen of the air, he inferred, had 'attenuated' or made less virulent the micro-organisms in the 'stale' culture. Why, then, he asked himself, could he not cultivate germs to any required degree of virulence or non-virulence? With these 'controlled' germs, he could induce an immunity, as in the inoculated fowl, to future infection.

From chickens, Pasteur turned his attention to sheep and cattle which, at that time, were all too liable in France and elsewhere to be attacked by the deadly disease known as anthrax or splenetic fever. Here, Pasteur discovered that the virulence of germs could be increased or lessened at will if the germs were introduced into the bodies of different living animals and then recovered, later, in fresh cultures taken from those animals. He had made one of the most momentous discoveries in the history of medicine.

There were those who ridiculed his opinions and cast doubts on his scientific honesty, but Pasteur soon routed all the sceptics by an experiment he carried out at the farm of Pouilly-le-Fort near Melun. In this classic demonstration, Pasteur took three flocks of sheep. The first group, of ten sheep, were to act as the 'control' animals. The second flock, of twenty-five sheep, had previously been inoculated with an attenuated culture of live anthrax germs. The third flock – also of twenty-five sheep – had not.

Then, before an audience of scientists, doctors and other interested parties, some of whom believed in the importance of what he was doing and some of whom did not, Pasteur injected all the animals save those in his control group with a virulent culture of anthrax germs. To the great satisfaction of his friends and sympathisers and to the equally great chagrin of his critics, all the uninoculated animals died, as he had said that they would, and all the inoculated ones remained alive.

The first human disease that Pasteur tried to prevent by inoculation was rabies, or hydrophobia – a disease which causes sufferers to die in dreadful agonies, and for which there is, to this day, no certain cure.

When Pasteur started his researches into hydrophobia – which, in humans, is associated particularly with dog bites – he was under the natural but mistaken impression that the relevant micro-organism would be found in the saliva of the

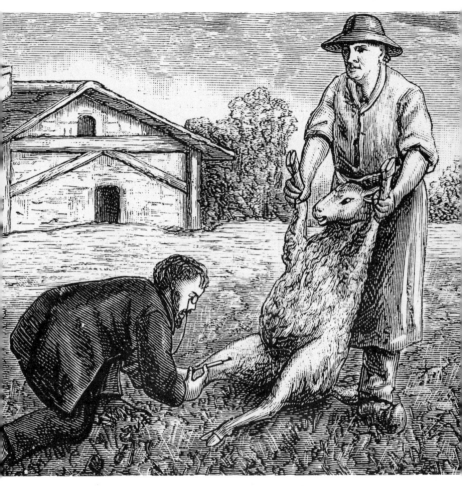

Pasteur inoculating a sheep against anthrax

animal that carried the infection. Then he found that he was
unable to transmit the disease to animals by inoculating them
with saliva taken from a human patient who was suffering
from hydrophobia. From that, and from the nature of the
principal symptoms of the disease, he inferred that the micro-
organisms that caused it would be found in the central
nervous system of the patient, whether human or animal.

Having established this, he was able to use the central nervous system of rabbits for growing the micro-organisms he needed. By drying, for varying lengths of time, the infected rabbits' spinal cords, Pasteur found that he could produce material for inoculation that would have its virulence attenuated to any degree he desired.

But then Pasteur ran into difficulties. There were nearly three million dogs in France, he found out, and it would have been quite impossible, for preventive purposes, to inoculate every one of them. So, he came to the conclusion that he would have to provide some form of treatment, instead, for human beings who had already been bitten by rabid dogs or other animals. In 1885, with immense courage and faith in his own judgment, Pasteur inoculated with increasing strengths of virus a young Alsatian boy named Joseph Meister who had been bitten in fourteen places by a rabid dog. The experiment was entirely successful and the boy was saved from a certain and very painful death. Pasteur's treatment for potential hydrophobia was adopted, after that, throughout the world, the first 'Pasteur Institute' being inaugurated in Paris in 1888.

Although the work done by Joseph Lister and Louis Pasteur during the nineteenth century entitles them to be numbered among the greatest benefactors of mankind, both would have been ready to admit how much they owed to the whole-hearted co-operation of other people. The elaborate antiseptic procedures that are seen, now, in the operating theatres of all civilised hospitals were developed slowly but certainly from Lister's earliest rituals. But it was William S. Halstead, of the Johns Hopkins Hospital, Baltimore, who first suggested, in 1889, that rubber gloves should be worn by surgeons and nurses. He intended, primarily, to protect the operators' hands from the powerful antiseptics in use at the time, but it soon became clear that the use of the gloves might also be of benefit to the patients. And, it was Johann von Miculicz of Breslau (now Wroclaw) who first recommended, in 1896, that gauze face-masks should be used. He did this after a bacteriologist colleague named Karl Flügge had found that even when one is speaking in a quiet voice innumerable tiny droplets containing bacteria are sent out into the air. Ernst von Bergmann, at Berlin, first suggested surgical sterilisation by steam.

Pasteur's great work on immunology could hardly have been carried out so swiftly and successfully if the German scientist Robert Koch (1834–1910) had not laid the foundations for all modern bacteriological techniques. It was Koch, for instance, who first showed how the anthrax bacillus could be grown and how it could be obtained unmixed with other organisms in a 'pure' culture. Koch showed, too, the advantages of growing the different kinds of bacteria on solid, rather than in liquid, media, and it was Koch who first demonstrated that varying micro-organisms could be distinguished from one another by the way they absorbed different dyes from solutions. From this developed the vitally important technique of 'staining' bacteria, which enables them to be seen more readily under the microscope and helps the bacteriologist to identify the different species.

Pasteur celebrated his seventieth birthday in 1892 – it was the year in which Lister reached the age of retirement and gave up his Chair and his hospital appointment. The two men met at the festivities held at the Sorbonne in honour of Pasteur. When Pasteur entered the assembly, leaning on the arm of President Carnot, it was Lister's privilege to hail him in this way:

> Truly, there does not exist in the wide world an individual to whom medical science owes more than to you.[8]

In his reply, Pasteur expressed the happiness he felt in seeing before him so many foreign delegates, since he believed that

> science and peace must triumph over ignorance and war, that nations will unite not to destroy but to instruct one another, and that the future will belong to those who have

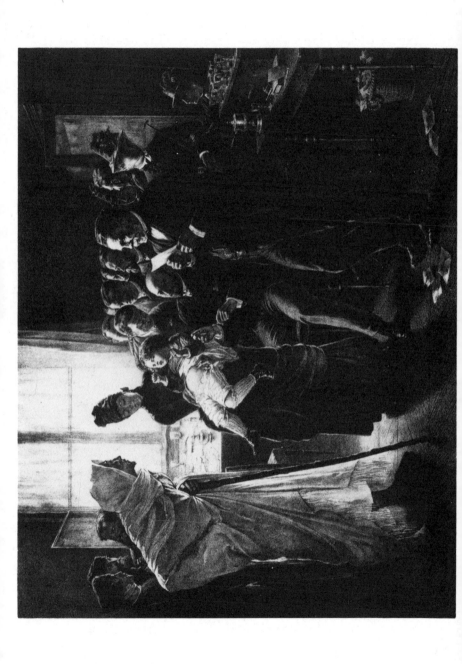

done most for suffering humanity. I refer to you, my dear Lister.[9]

After his retirement, Lister's days were filled with public duties. In 1895 he was made President of the Royal Society and, in 1896, President of the British Association. He was involved in the affairs of several other eminent bodies – and honours were heaped upon him. In 1897 he was given a peerage, and five years later he became one of the original members of the Order of Merit, which was instituted to mark the Coronation of King Edward VII. His eightieth birthday, in 1907, was celebrated with the greatest respect in many different parts of the world. By that time, though, his health had started to fail, and he was living in retirement at Walmer, in Kent, when, five years later, the end came. Among the countless tributes paid to Lister in the days that followed his death there was one especially moving eulogy, made on behalf of the Royal College of Surgeons, which contained these words: 'His gentle nature, imperturbable temper, resolute will, indifference to ridicule, and tolerance of hostile criticism combined to make him one of the noblest of men. His work will last for all time; humanity will bless him evermore and his fame will be immortal.'[10]

# 7

# Birth and Infancy
# in the Nineteenth Century

*. . . Once more unto the breach, dear friends . . .*

WILLIAM SHAKESPEARE, *King Henry V*

At the end of the eighteenth century, two-thirds of the children born in the Metropolitan Area of London died before they were five years old. According to William Buchan's *Domestic Medicine*, published in 1784: 'It appears from the annual register of the dead that almost one half of the children born in Great Britain die under twelve years of age.'

Women, at that time, sought treatment in hospitals only if they were forced to, through poverty, illegitimacy, or obstetrical complications.[1] By the end of the nineteenth century, safe and relatively painless childbirth could be looked forward to by the vast majority of expectant mothers, whether they had their babies in hospital or in their homes.

One of the greatest changes came in the capacity of midwives, and in the attitude of officials and members of the public to them. During the eighteenth century, a typical midwife would be at the best semi-skilled. She – at that time there were only a few man midwives – would work, normally, in a grossly overheated room and she and her assistants would usually be in an advanced state of intoxication.

In the early years of the nineteenth century, many medical men were urging that midwives should be officially recognised and properly instructed, but these innovators made little progress against their more conservative colleagues. Then, in 1812, the officials of the Society of Apothecaries made an appeal to Parliament for the recognition of midwives and a petition was presented, but the Members of Parliament were so prejudiced against midwives that the Committee of the House of Commons would not allow the name to be mentioned. A little later, Charles Dickens inadvertently increased the unpopularity of midwives by creating Sairey Gamp and Betsey Prig. With the best of intentions, he had hoped to draw to the public view the type of person most often entrusted with the care of the sick and of females in labour.

Then, in 1864, a Ladies' Obstetrical College was founded in London, the aim of the college being to introduce educated women such as the daughters of medical men and clergymen into the midwifery service and to provide them with proper facilities for learning the theory and practice of midwifery.

In 1866 Dr. Farr, Superintendent of the Statistical Department in the Office of the Registrar General, undertook to investigate a report on the causes of infant mortality. One recommendation of the report was that an Examining Board should be set up so that potential midwives might be tested and granted a Diploma of Proficiency. The first examination was held in 1872, under the auspices of the London Obstetrical Society, which had been founded in 1858. The qualifications required by the Society for those who wished to sit this examination were: they had to be at least twenty-one years old, and not over thirty; they had to provide a certificate of moral character; they had to provide proof of having attended no fewer than twenty-five cases under supervision that satisfied the Board of Examiners; and they had to provide proof of having attended a course of approved lectures. Last of all, they had to undergo a written and an oral examination. Six candidates only, from the whole of the Metropolis, presented themselves for the final ordeals.

During the dying decades of the nineteenth century, several lying-in hospitals began to train midwives and to issue certificates of proficiency. From 1872 onwards, the

General Medical Council made great efforts to secure State recognition of midwives. In 1881 the Midwives' Institute was set up with the object of obtaining for midwives some form of that recognition. The first Bill was unsuccessfully introduced to Parliament in 1890, and a further seven Bills were introduced, also unsuccessfully, after that. It was not until 1902 that a ninth Bill passed all stages and received the Royal Assent. The 1902 Act was known as 'an Act to secure the better training and supervision of midwives'.

In the hot, sweaty, unventilated rooms in which the early nineteenth-century midwives performed their duties, child-bed fever, or puerperal infection, provided a constant menace. It was still, at the time, the scourge of maternity hospitals in all parts of Europe, the mortality rate in many of these hospitals being as high as 25 or 30 per cent. Steps to combat the disease had been taken by Doctor Charles White of Manchester (born 1728) and Doctor Alexander Gordon of Aberdeen, but it was Ignaz Phillip Semmelweis who devised the first really hygienic techniques ever used in midwifery. Semmelweis has been called 'The Saviour of Mothers', for his innovations may be truly said to have opened a new era in medical science.

Semmelweis was born in Buda, Hungary, on 1 July 1818, and was educated at the Universities of Pest and Vienna. Having been awarded a doctor's degree by Vienna in 1844, he was appointed assistant at the obstetric clinic in that city. He soon became concerned with the problem of puerperal fever. Several possible causes of the infection were being suggested. It was induced by overcrowding, thought some, or by poor ventilation. Others blamed the onset of lactation, calling this 'miasma'. Semmelweis set himself to investigate scientifically the cause of childbed fever against strong opposition from his chief who, like most other European physicians, was convinced that the disease could never be prevented.

Semmelweis's first really important discovery came when he noticed that the death rate from childbed fever was two or three times higher in one division of the clinic than it was in the other. In most respects the divisions were identical but, he observed, students were trained in the apparently dangerous division while midwives were trained in the division that seemed relatively safe. So he decided that something unknown was almost certainly being handed on, by the students, to the women they examined in labour. His views were confirmed when one of his friends died after contracting an infected wound while examining a woman who had died of puerperal fever. It seemed, then, that students who moved from the dissecting room to the maternity ward might be carrying with them some infection that they had acquired from mothers who had died of the disease. To many of the healthy mothers, this mysterious evil was proving fatal.

Semmelweis's next step was of historic importance: he instructed all the students to bathe their hands in a solution of chlorinated lime before they ventured to examine any patient. The results of this order were spectacular: the mortality rates in the division visited by the students fell from over 18 per cent to under two per cent, and in two of the months of 1848 no patient at all died in childbirth in the division. The results of Semmelweis's innovation were greeted enthusiastically by the younger medical men of Vienna. Some of the older, more conservative doctors were less appreciative, however, Semmelweis's director being among the most obdurate.

During the year 1848, Semmelweis became involved in political activities in Vienna, and he soon found that his work for the liberal cause made his professional opponents even more hostile to him than they had been before. In the following year he was asked to give up his job at the clinic. He applied for a post at the University of Vienna which would mean that he could continue to teach midwifery, but he was rejected. Next, he lectured to the Medical Society of Vienna on puerperal fever and its origins, and his talk was warmly received. Encouraged by this, he applied again for the University post. On this occasion he was successful, but a number of humiliating restrictions were imposed on him, to which he felt unable to submit. So he quitted Vienna in 1850 and returned to Pest.

For the next six years, Semmelweis worked at the St Rochus Hospital in Pest. When a serious epidemic of puerperal fever broke out, he was put in charge of the obstetrics wards and, using the methods he had found so successful in Vienna, he managed to reduce the mortality rate until its yearly average was below one per cent. In 1861, he published a book in which he expounded his ideas. He sent copies of it to many leading obstetricians and to medical societies in a number of countries, but his ideas were, in general, considered too advanced, and most of his readers rejected them. The Editor of the Journal of the Medical Association of Vienna even wrote that it was 'time to stop all this nonsense about the chlorine hand wash'. Wearied in spirit by all this opposition, Semmelweis broke down completely and had to be taken to a mental hospital where he died of an infection that he had contracted while he was operating, before he became ill. His ideas were afterwards generally accepted by the medical profession, Joseph Lister paying him this special tribute: 'I think with the greatest admiration of him and his achievement and it fills me with joy that at last he is given the respect due to him'.

Also to be feared by many expectant mothers in the nineteenth century was eclampsia – a severe form of toxaemia encountered in pregnancy and characterised by convulsions similar to those of epilepsy. The fits are exhausting, and if they recur frequently heart failure may develop, or the woman may have a cerebral haemorrhage. Inhalation of blood or mucus may lead to pneumonia. Any of these complications may prove fatal.

It was the Russian obstetrician Stroganoff who made, in the late nineteenth century, two important observations and based his treatment on them. He realised that the fewer fits one of his patients had, the more likely she was to recover. He noticed, too, that any disturbance – noise, bright lights, or too sudden movement or activity – could start off a fit. So he kept his patients absolutely quiet and undisturbed in an almost noiseless environment. He made his nurses wear quiet slippers and unstarched aprons and he urged them to converse only in whispers. He prescribed for his patients generous doses of powerful drugs such as morphine and chloral, which so dulled their senses that the processes of nursing and even the contractions of labour hardly roused them. This treatment was remarkably successful, and even today the management of eclampsia is based, in general, on Stroganoff's recommendations. It is not now a very common trouble, occuring in Britain only once in about a thousand births.

Once safely born, a baby at the end of the nineteenth century would have had a much better chance of surviving infancy than a child of similar age in the early 1800s. The custom of 'swaddling' infants in tight, restricting clothes had virtually disappeared during the century, under the influence of a number of pioneers who had encouraged lighter, freer coverings. The use of powerful drugs such as laudanum to quieten babies had gradually been discontinued, too, though inquests in 1837–8 had still shown that fifty-two infants out of a total of a hundred and eighty-six had perished, primarily, through the administration of opium. The rubber nipple, patented in 1845, had solved many of the problems of feeding away from the breast; and substances much more suitable than 'pap' (bread or flour soaked in milk or in water) were being used as food, largely due to the lead given by the great German chemist Justus von Liebig.

Liebig (1803–73) devoted most of the last thirty-five years of his life to investigating the chemistry of the processes of life, both animal and vegetable. During his researches, he classified the various articles of food eaten by humans in accordance with the special function performed by each in the economy of the body. Contrary to most of the informed thought of the time, he taught that the heat of the body is the result of the processes of combustion and oxidisation performed within the organism. In the course of his investigations, he evolved a preparation which was, as nearly as he could achieve this aim, a perfectly balanced food for infants. This, with Liebig's 'Extract of Meat', for which he also vouched, quickly became world-famous.

# 8

# Going to Hospital
# in the Nineteenth Century

*. . . A soldier of the Legion lay dying in Algiers –*
*There was lack of woman's nursing, there was dearth of woman's tears . . .*

CAROLINE ELIZABETH SARAH NORTON (1808–77)
*Bingen on the Rhine*

Going to hospital in the early nineteenth century was an experience to be avoided at all costs. No sick or injured person who could possibly be nursed at home or in a medical man's private residence would choose, in preference, to enter the squalid and crowded wards of the public institutions. We can get some idea from the notes compiled by Florence Nightingale a little later in the century of the terrible conditions that had to be endured by those who, by poverty or through force of circumstance, were compelled to take refuge in these dirty and foul-smelling places:

The floors were made of ordinary wood which, owing to lack of cleaning and lack of sanitary conveniences for the patients' use, had become "saturated with organic matter, which when washed give off the smell of something quite other than soap and water". Walls and ceilings were "of common plaster" also "saturated with impurity". Heating was supplied by a single fire at the end of each ward, and in winter windows were kept closed for warmth, sometimes for months at a time. In some hospitals half the windows were boarded up in winter. After a time the smell became "sickening", walls streamed with moisture, and a "minute vegetation appeared". The remedy for this was "frequent lime washing with scraping", but the workmen engaged on the task "frequently became seriously ill" . . .[1]

Into each of these insanitary wards as many beds would be crowded as possible – to have fifty or even sixty patients in a single ward would have been looked on, then, as sound and economical hospital management. The fact that many, if not the majority, of the patients would have come from the filthy and cholera-ridden slums that abounded at the time, and would have been chronically dirty, cannot have made a stay in hospital any more tolerable for the normally fastidious. Florence Nightingale also had some pungent comments to make on this aspect of early nineteenth-century hospitalisation:

> The nurses did not as a general rule wash patients, they could *never* wash their feet – and it was with difficulty and only in great haste that they could have a drop of water, just to *dab* their hands and face. The beds on which the patients lay were dirty. It was common practice to put a new patient into the same sheets used by the last occupant of the bed, and mattresses were generally of flock, sodden and seldom if ever cleaned.[2]

Condemned to stay in these wretched conditions, a typical patient of the time might well turn to gin or brandy as the only readily available placebo. No serious attempt would ever be made to keep alcoholic 'medicines' out of the wards; why, ran the argument, should not a patient be allowed to drift into a state of near-oblivion, obtaining thereby at least a temporary relief from his or her sufferings? The noise in most hospital wards was invariably deafening. Drunken patients would quarrel constantly and would frequently fight with one another. Representatives of the Law – who were not, usually, at that time, very authoritative or very efficient – would have to be called in to restore some kind of order. It is hard to see how the less heavily intoxicated patients managed to get any sleep at all.

The women employed to 'nurse' the patients in these Rabelaisian surroundings would be drawn exclusively from the very lowest classes of the community – who else could be persuaded to take on such a miserable and ill-rewarded task? – and they would almost invariably be slatternly and disreputable. 'The nurses are all drunkards, sisters and all', reported one of the physicians attached to a large London hospital in 1851, 'and there are but two nurses whom the surgeons can trust to give the patients their medicine'.[3] Three years later, the head nurse of a London hospital told Florence Nightingale that 'in the course of her large experience she had never known a nurse who was not drunken, and there was immoral conduct practised in the very wards, of which she gave me some awful examples'.[4]

Florence Nightingale, who was to do more than anyone else to change the appalling conditions in British hospitals (and, as her influence grew, in the hospitals of many other parts of the world), came from a comfortable, sheltered upper-middle-class background. She was born in the early summer of 1820 in Florence, where her parents happened to be living. There was already one child in the Nightingale nursery: Florence's elder sister Parthe, who grew up to regard the younger girl as a conveniently clever person who had no right to devote her energies to anyone else but Parthe. The family returned to England in 1821 and the rest of Florence's childhood was spent, in consequence, in the well-appointed houses that her father and mother purchased and the equally luxurious homes of their numerous relatives and friends.

But Florence's childhood was, in other respects, by no means normal. While she was still quite young, she became convinced that she was in some way different from other people, and this obsession with her own individuality made her shy, stubborn and given to ill-natured outbursts of feeling. Even before she was seven years old – she recorded later – she had decided that the comfortable and leisurely way of living of her family was utterly distasteful to her. She had been born, she found it plain, for Higher Things.

Until she was shown exactly what the Higher Things were to be, Florence laboured conscientiously at her lessons, studying French, German, Greek, Italian, History, Latin and Philosophy with her father. Her father taught her because no governess could be found who would be as well-bred and refined as Mrs Nightingale would expect, while being, at the same time, intellectually capable of instructing such an unusual child. The leisure-time activities normally prescribed for young ladies of her class – embroidery, paying social calls with Mama, and 'doing the flowers' – bored Florence literally to tears.

Then, in February 1837, when she was not quite seventeen, and when her family were making preparations for an extended tour in Europe, this earnest young woman heard the voice of God speaking to her. He did not speak to her quietly through her conscience, as the phrase is usually meant to suggest. He spoke to her loudly and clearly and she listened to Him with rapt attention in exactly the same way as the Maid of Orleans had listened to her 'voices' when she was approximately the same age as Florence. From that time on, Florence Nightingale knew with absolute certainty that she had been instructed to devote her life to some form of Divine service.

Unfortunately, though, God had omitted to tell her, or even to hint at, the form that that service should take. The idea that it might have anything to do with nursing the sick was not to occur to her for several more years. Meanwhile, she recorded in a private note her conviction that if she were worthy to be God's servant she would have to overcome the temptation to 'shine in Society'.[5] She was sufficiently intelligent, good-looking and attractive to have done so if she had not been discouraged by the Divine message she had received.

By 1842, which was a year of dire economic distress in England, Florence Nightingale had become personally involved in the social work that was being undertaken at that time by many of the well-to-do, if not through goodness of heart, at least as a form of insurance against the possibility of revolution. Visiting the sick and starving cottagers in the villages near her family homes, she became fully aware for the first time of the wretched, overcrowded and insanitary conditions in which the underprivileged people of her generation were forced to live. 'My mind is absorbed with the idea of the sufferings of man', she wrote in a private note in the summer of that year. 'It besets me behind and before, a very one-sided view, but I can hardly see anything else and all that poets sing of the glories of this world seems to me untrue. All the people I see are eaten up with care or poverty or disease'.[6]

In the autumn of 1842, Florence Nightingale called on the Prussian Ambassador, the Chevalier Bunsen, with whom she had previously become friendly, and who happened to be liberal-minded as well as extremely wealthy. 'What can a person like myself do to lift the load of suffering from the helpless and the miserable?'[7] she asked the Chevalier. The Chevalier, who much admired Miss Nightingale, told her of a Pastor Fliedner and his wife who were doing some excellent work at Kaiserwerth on the Rhine. At Kaiserwerth, he said, there was a Protestant institution which had a hospital attached to it. In this hospital, the Fliedners had been training a number of deaconesses to nurse the invalid and wounded poor. Florence Nightingale listened but she does not seem to have thought of herself, at that stage, as a possible nurse.

In the following year, however, she started to spend an increasing amount of time in poor people's homes – nursing them, and trying to get their lives properly organised. The Nightingale parents – sympathetic at first, because they were generous-hearted – became, later, deeply concerned with what they regarded as their daughter's 'unnatural' interest in the sick poor and they did everything they possibly could to win her back to more conventional activities.

By the summer of 1844, more than seven years after

Florence Nightingale had first heard the voice of God calling her to His service, the dedicated young woman had found out for certain the nature of the work that her Maker had intended for her. She asked a visitor from America – the philanthropist Doctor Gridley Howe, who had founded in Boston an Institute for the Blind – if he thought that it would be unsuitable and unbecoming for a young Englishwoman to devote herself to works of charity in hospitals and elsewhere as Catholic sisters did. Would it be, she asked, a dreadful thing? Doctor Howe gave her the answer that she had been hoping to hear: 'My dear Miss Florence, it would be unusual, and in England whatever is unusual is thought to be unsuitable; but I say to you "Go forward", if you have a vocation for that way of life, act up to your inspiration and you will find there is never anything unbecoming or unladylike in doing your duty for the good of others. Choose, go on with it, wherever it may lead you and God be with you'.[8]

Before the end of that year, Florence Nightingale had proposed to her family that she should be allowed to spend three months in the Infirmary at Salisbury to learn the techniques – such as they were at that time – of nursing. The principal physician of the hospital, a Dr Fowler, was an old friend of the family, and if her plan had been accepted Florence Nightingale would have been able to stay, during her training, in the Fowlers' respectable and comfortable home. But the plan was not accepted. Her mother became furious; her sister became hysterical; her father let her know, more quietly, that he was disgusted. Eight more years had to elapse before Florence Nightingale was able to follow, openly, her vocation.

Those eight years were years of suffering and frustration so acute that Florence Nightingale was driven, at times, to the verge of a breakdown. But the years were not entirely wasted for, without bringing her activities too forcibly to the notice of her family, Miss Nightingale set herself the task of finding out, by laborious enquiries and correspondence, as much as she possibly could about the different ways in which hospitals were organised in various parts of the world, and she gained a small reputation as an expert in this unfashionable subject. She enlarged her circle of friends, too, and the members of one family with whom she became especially intimate – the Herberts of Wilton – were to be particularly important to her when, at last, she decided to take her destiny into her own hands and to escape from the influence of her domineering and possessive relations.

When, once, she had escaped from them temporarily, she had managed to reach the Institution at Kaiserwerth and had spent a short time there inspecting the work of the deaconesses, but while she had been deeply impressed by the piety of everyone there she had not been so impressed by the general hygiene. On her first really independent travels, made when she had already reached the age of thirty-two, she headed for Paris, where she spent a month visiting hospitals and other institutions. In the course of her visits she watched many patients being examined by the doctors and she was present at a number of operations. She had intended, at the end of the month, to enter the hospital of the Sisters of Charity in the Rue Oudinot, to submit herself to a course of training in their systems of nursing, but before she could do so she heard that her grandmother was seriously ill and she returned to England to look after the old lady during her last days.

Meanwhile, Florence Nightingale's friends, who knew and approved of her break with her immediate relations, had been looking on her behalf for some form of employment that might suit her. Early in April 1853 one of them heard that an obscure establishment known as the Institution for the Care of Sick Gentlewomen in Distressed Circumstances, which had been sadly running down, was to be reorganised by the committee of charitably minded persons who were responsible for its upkeep. To supervise this reorganisation, the members of the committee required a suitable Superintendent. The friend of Florence Nightingale suggested that

Miss Nightingale might be the person for whom they were looking. Florence Nightingale, who was to refer to the place later as 'a Sanatorium for Sick Governesses run by a Committee of Fine Ladies', was duly approached and interviewed by the Fine Ladies. She became involved in protracted negotiations with them, in the course of which she made it plain that unless she were given by the Fine Ladies a completely free hand to reorganise the Institution in the way she thought best, she would have nothing to do with it. The Fine Ladies were impressed by Miss Nightingale's quiet air of competence and by her determination, but they were a little worried by the fact that she came from such a superior social class. Was it proper, they wondered, for someone who was a 'Lady' to nurse someone else who was not a 'Lady'? They were more concerned still when they heard reports that Miss Nightingale's nearest and dearest female relatives had kicked up a tremendous fuss when they had found out that Miss Nightingale was even considering taking such a post, and that other members of her family had been publicly declaring that she was 'lowering herself' by 'going into service'. With the steely resolve which was to become internationally renowned, Miss Nightingale managed to reduce all these little local difficulties to entirely manageable proportions. She even managed to persuade her father, who had been deeply shocked by the feminine quarrels which had rent his immediate family circle, and who had retreated, in consequence, into the impregnable masculine confines of the Athenaeum Club, to write a letter to the members of the Fine Ladies' committee in which he said that he 'approved' of what his daughter Florence was doing.

By the end of April 1853 Florence Nightingale had been appointed to the post of Superintendent of the new Institution. She was to receive no financial remuneration of any kind for her duties. This did not matter to her too much as her father was by that time giving her a comfortable allowance. But she had also agreed to pay, out of her own pocket, all the expenses that would accrue from the engagement of a 'superior elderly respectable person'[9] who would act as her Matron and Housekeeper, and whose advanced age would help to compensate, in the eyes of the world, for Miss Nightingale's own lack of maturity.

The building chosen for the Institution in its new guise – Number One, Harley Street – needed to have innumerable alterations and improvements done to it before it would be anything like good enough for the exacting Miss Nightingale. The Superintendent-elect, visiting the Catholics in Paris in a renewed attempt to undergo training as a nurse, was struck down with measles, and from her sick bed in the cell of a *Soeur de la Charité* and from a convalescent's couch in the more luxurious drawing-room of a friend sent long, carefully detailed instructions to the members of the London committee. Most of the suggestions she made may seem to us, now, all too obvious. She wanted a 'windlass installation' or lift, for instance, so that the patients' meals could be taken speedily and conveniently upstairs from the kitchens; and she wanted a system of bells by which patients in trouble could attract the attention of the relevant nurse. When she returned to London from Paris she found that all her directives had been disregarded and that virtually nothing had been done. So she herself had to set to and work like a whirlwind. On 20 August 1853 she wrote to a friend:

> I have had to prepare this immense house for patients in ten days – without a bit of help but only hindrance from my committee. I have been 'in service' ten days and have had to furnish an entirely empty house in that time. We take in patients this Monday and have not got our workmen out yet. From Committees, Charity and Schism, from the Church of England, from philanthropy and all deceits of the devil, Good Lord deliver us.[10]

Even before the first patients were admitted to the Institution, the members of the committee who had engaged Florence Nightingale were painfully aware that they had taken on a tartar. To their amazement, they found that she insisted that other patients should be admitted, besides those who belonged to the Established Church of England. She insisted, too, that these other non-Protestant patients should be visited, when they wished and needed to be, by their own priests, muftis or rabbis, though the members of the committee insisted in their turn that these dangerous intruders should be met at the door by Miss Nightingale and escorted by her to and from the beds of those they had come to visit in case they attempted to proselytise. But the quiet young lady proved to have a perfect genius for organisation, and before six months had passed the Institution was running so smoothly that Miss Nightingale could refer to it disparagingly as 'this little mole hill'.[11]

Miss Nightingale's energetic rule at the Institution resulted in such drastic innovations as the substitution of home-made jams for 'bought' jams. They were so much cheaper, she found; the preserves made in the Institution's own kitchen cost less than a third of the cost of those that had been purchased in the shops. And an elderly clergyman was appointed to the post of Chaplain to the Institution in place of a younger and more presentable curate who had shown a dangerous inclination to flirt with Miss Nightingale's young ladies. These and similar changes were hardly of monumental significance, but they provided Miss Nightingale with the practical experience she badly needed before she could become a wholly successful administrator on a very much larger scale.

Miss Nightingale's move on to a more important scene might never have been made if the landing of the Allied armies in the Crimean peninsula in the autumn of 1854 had not been, administratively, a disaster from the word 'Go'. The trouble stemmed, in the first place, from the fact that when the British Army tried to embark at Varna for the Crimea, the Army's officers found that there were not enough transport vessels available to carry all the necessary fighting men and all their necessary equipment. So most of the necessary equipment was jettisoned. Bedding, stores, and the regimental medicine chests were all left behind. On 14 September, the fighting men disembarked at a place which had the ominous name 'Calamity Bay'. Hundreds of the men were suffering from cholera and were in no state to fight anyone. 'My God!' exploded the Staff Surgeon of the Light Division. 'They have landed this army without any kind of hospital transport, litters or carts or anything'. The army advanced towards the enemy; achieved at Alma, a week later, a resounding victory; and then had to suffer, with entirely inadequate resources, the appalling consequences of a major military engagement.

The aftermath of that victory was described by William Howard Russell, Special War Correspondent of *The Times*, in a historic series of dispatches:

> Not only are there not sufficient surgeons . . . Not only are there no dressers and nurses . . . There is not even linen to make bandages . . . Can it be said that the battle of the Alma has been an event to take the world by surprise? Yet . . . there is no preparation for the commonest surgical operations! Not only are the men kept, in some cases for a week, without the hand of a medical man coming near their wounds, not only are they left to expire in agony, unheeded and shaken off, though catching desperately at the surgeon as he makes his rounds through the fetid ship, but now . . . it is found that the commonest appliances of a workhouse sick ward are wanting, and that the men must die through the medical staff of the British Army having forgotten that old rags are necessary for the dressing of wounds.[2]

The people who read *The Times*, back in Britain, had been thinking of the war in the Crimea entirely in terms of glamorous confrontations, heroic charges and desperate acts of bravery. When they learned from their favourite morning paper that the wounded and the sick, who had been taken back after a terrible journey over the Black Sea to Scutari, were lying on the floors of the Barrack Hospital there because there were no beds, and were being given no food because there were no kitchens in the hospital, they were understandably a little disturbed. They would have been even more disturbed, they might even have been driven to some desperate form of action, if they could actually have been transported to Scutari and could have seen the mangled soldiers lying on the hospital floors covered only with dirty blood-soaked and pus-caked blankets. Cholera was raging through the wards and there was ordure everywhere. There was no water with which the tormented men might be cleaned. There were no vessels in which any water, if available, could have been carried to the wards. To have asked for pure water so that a man in agony could have a relieving drink would have been like asking, at that time, for a few ounces of the moon.

At once, letters poured in on the Editor of *The Times*, and one of them, which asked 'Why have we no Sisters of Charity?', was seen by Sidney Herbert, the Secretary at War, who was one of Florence Nightingale's closest friends. On 15 October he wrote to Miss Nightingale suggesting that she should go to Scutari at the head of a party of nurses. The expedition would have the Government's full approval and backing, he added, and all the expenses of the exercise would be officially defrayed.

To Florence Nightingale, Sidney Herbert's plan came as no great surprise. She had, in fact, already arranged to set off for the war front with a small party of nurses, and was due to leave in a few days' time, the necessary financing having been undertaken, in the main, by a wealthy and pious widow named Lady Maria Forester. Miss Nightingale had not ventured to tell the Secretary at War of her plans because she knew how harassed he must have been by the trenchant criticisms that were being showered, from almost every side, on his undeserving head. Being asked to act officially on the Government's behalf gave Miss Nightingale a lot more scope, though, and she immediately consented to co-operate with the Minister at War, on condition that the Committee of Ladies which had engaged her to administer the Harley Street Institution would consent to her leaving the place, at least temporarily, in other hands. Sidney Herbert, she gathered, was in a quite optimistic frame of mind:

> You will have seen in the papers that there is a great deficiency of nurses at the Hospital at Scutari [he had written to her].
>
> The other alleged deficiencies, namely of medical men, lint, sheets, etc., must, if they have really ever existed, have been remedied ere this, as the number of medical officers with the Army amounted to one to every 95 men in the whole force, being nearly double what we have ever had before, and 30 more surgeons went out 3 weeks ago, and would by this time, therefore, be at Constantinople. A further supply went on Thursday, and a fresh batch sail next week.
>
> As to medical stores, they have been sent out in profusion; lint by the ton weight, 15,000 pairs of sheets, medicine, wine, arrowroot in the same proportion; and the only way of accounting for the deficiency at Scutari, if it exists, is that the mass of stores went to Varna, and was not sent back when the Army left for the Crimea; but four days would have remedied this. In the meanwhile fresh stores are arriving.
>
> But the deficiency of female nurses is undoubted, none but male nurses having ever been admitted to military hospitals.
>
> It would be impossible to carry about a large staff of female nurses with the Army in the field. But at Scutari, having now a fixed hospital, no military reason exists against their introduction, and I am confident they might be introduced with great benefit, for hospital orderlies must be very rough hands, and most of them, on such an occasion as this, very inexperienced ones.
>
> I receive numbers of offers from ladies to go out, but

they are ladies who have no conception of what an hospital is, nor of the nature of its duties; and they would, when the time came, either recoil from the work or be entirely useless, and consequently – what is worse – entirely in the way. Nor would these ladies probably ever understand the necessity, especially in a military hospital, of strict obedience to rule.[13]

Florence Nightingale made the necessary preparations for her journey with almost incredible speed. She allowed four days only for engaging nurses – forty of them, she and Sidney Herbert agreed, if such a number of suitable persons could be found; for fitting them out with uniforms – she was insistent on that – and for making all the arrangements for their travel. Her friends sped to all parts of London in a hectic search for clean, sober, competent women who could be induced by offers of wages that were nearly double those paid in the London hospitals, to submit themselves to Miss Nightingale's absolute authority and to agree to obey the strict rules she laid down concerning the proper conduct of nurses. Only fourteen people were discovered who had any previous experience of working in hospitals and who would accept this daunting assignment. Another two dozen inexperienced people drawn from a variety of religious institutions were engaged in circumstances that would have driven any person less resolute than Florence Nightingale to despair. 'Fat drunken old dames of fourteen stone and over must be barred', she was to order later, from Scutari. 'The provision of bedsteads is not strong enough'.[14]

The arrival of Miss Nightingale's party at Scutari would have been an upsetting experience even if many members of the expeditionary force, including the leader herself, had not been seriously weakened by prolonged bouts of sea sickness. As the distressed females tottered off the picturesque painted boats in which they had been ferried across the Bosphorus they saw, in the water by the tumbledown landing stage, the bloated body of a large grey horse which was being rudely buffeted by the tide, while a pack of starving dogs fought with each other for the chance to sink their fangs into it. The sloping ground that led from the landing stage to the hospital was slippery with mud and ordure and littered with rubbish of all kinds. As the band of women from England made their way through the wide and high gateway of the Barrack Hospital they were so depressed that over the door, Miss Nightingale said, could well have been written 'Abandon hope all ye who enter here'. It is salutary to recall some of the worst hardships that these women had then to endure.

They had to face, first, the hostility of the doctors already working at Scutari who believed, in the words of the Army Medical Department, that female nurses in a military hospital were 'an unwise indulgence unfavourable to military discipline and to the recovery of the patients'. With one single exception those doctors intended to ignore Miss Nightingale and the nurses she had brought from England. Any offers she might make to help with the work in the hospital would, they agreed, be coldly ignored. Miss Nightingale countered this by telling her nurses that under no circumstances whatsoever was any of them to enter a ward unless she had been specifically invited to do so by one or more of the doctors. Miss Nightingale's ban was strictly enforced, and her frustrated nurses were kept away from the patients they were eager to help for more than a fortnight. Then, as a result of further disastrous military operations, sick and wounded soldiers started to pour into the Scutari Hospital in such appalling numbers that the doctors were forced, willy-nilly, to forget their prejudices and to turn to Miss Nightingale and her band of females for assistance in what was, clearly, a desperate emergency.

The shortage of equipment in the hospital must have seemed to Miss Nightingale almost as amazing as the reception she was given by the medical men. The people who were responsible for ordering the equipment were invariably working at cross purposes with the people who had been given the job of obtaining it, and the Army's old-fashioned administrative systems were so inadequate that no one would have been able to act effectively on his own initiative, even if he had dared. So the men lay on the floors without proper bedding and, in a great many instances, without even shirts to cover their nakedness. There was virtually no furniture. There were no medical supplies. There was no table that could be used satisfactorily by the surgeons for the numerous operations that they were compelled to carry out, under the most daunting and dangerous conditions. There were no screens to hide the surgeons, at their work, from their future victims. There were plenty of rats, lice and fleas, but there were very few knives, forks or spoons. Miss Nightingale and her nurses, who were allowed just one pint of water per person per day for washing and drinking and for making tea, were comparatively lucky in that they had, each, a small tin bowl. But these vessels had to be used for a number of different purposes including feeding and the washing of faces and hands, so it is easy to see that the ladies' own personal circumstances were hardly hygienic.

The stench in that hospital must have been overpowering. Miss Nightingale estimated that there were at least a thousand men in the wards who were suffering from acute diarrhoea and there were fewer than two dozen chamber pots that they could use. There were tubs in the wards that the orderlies would usually refuse to empty. The privies were useless, because they could not be flushed, and liquid filth an inch deep on the floors around would have discouraged the barefooted men from attempting to reach them anyway. 'We have erysipelas, fever and gangrene', commented Miss Nightingale on these appalling conditions. 'The dysentery cases have died at the rate of one in two. The mortality of the operations is frightful'.[15]

Once she and her nurses were allowed to move freely into the wards, Florence Nightingale tackled with implacable determination the serious problems set by the inadequacies of the Scutari Hospital and by the administrative incapacity of the appointed officials. Because no one had ever been officially made responsible for getting the privies cleared and put into working order again, they would have continued in a disgusting state indefinitely if Miss Nightingale, with money to spend and the authority to spend it, had not taken the necessary steps to have them repaired. Because those responsible for supplying the hospital with goods of various kinds had been compelled, by military precedent, to send back to England for them, no goods of any consequence had appeared at Scutari and might never have appeared there if Miss Nightingale had not been able to draw on the funds contributed by the readers of *The Times* and by her own friends, and if she had not had the enterprise to act as the hospital's only effective purchasing officer. She refused to send back to England for anything if it could be bought locally, or in Constantinople which was, after all, one of the world's busiest trading centres. Within two months of her arrival at Scutari, Miss Nightingale – or her representatives – had purchased several cartloads of bedding, tables, forms, cutlery, clocks, pails, soap and scrubbing brushes, screens, trays and other necessities; and she had supplied, when the Medical Officers had asked for them for the men, approximately six thousand shirts, two thousand socks and five hundred pairs of drawers. 'I am a kind of General Dealer', she wrote to Sidney Herbert early in January 1855, 'in socks, shirts, knives and forks, wooden spoons, tin baths, tables and forms, cabbages and carrots, operating tables, towels and soap, small tooth combs, precipitate for destroying lice, scissors, bed pans and stump pillows'.[16]

As she laboured, almost without having a chance to sleep, in her dual roles of Superintendent of Female Nurses and Chief Purchasing Officer of the Hospital, Florence Nightingale aroused, in most of those she was required to oversee and of those she was required to serve, extraordinarily powerful feelings of love and admiration, but she was also fated to arouse, in certain lesser breasts, feelings of resentment and even of bitter hostility. The arrival at Scutari of a party of forty-six nurses which had been collected in London and dispatched to the Crimea without reference to Miss Nightingale angered the Lady Superintendent so mightily that she wrote a white-hot letter of protest to Sidney Herbert in which she threatened to resign immediately and to return to England forthwith. But Miss Nightingale was irreplaceable, and everyone knew it. Soon, presents from Queen Victoria started to arrive at the Scutari Hospital and were accompanied by a personal message from the Sovereign to Miss Nightingale, requiring Miss Nightingale to be made aware

> that your goodness and self devotion in giving yourself up to the soothing attendance upon these wounded and sick soldiers had been observed by the Queen with sentiments of the highest approval and admiration.[17]

Miss Nightingale's personal prestige was enhanced by this so enormously that no one at Scutari, however puffed up they may have happened to be, would have dared to question her authority. As the Queen had asked, further, that Miss Nightingale should suggest something that the Queen could do 'to testify her sense of the courage and endurance so abundantly shown by her sick soldiers'[18] Miss Nightingale was put into a very enviable position. She was able, after that, to write directly to the Queen, telling Her Majesty more or less exactly what she – Miss Nightingale – knew should be done. Why, for instance, should a soldier incapacitated by sickness contracted on the battlefield be paid less per day, while he was in hospital, than a soldier laid low by a battlefield injury? It was most unfair! Surely the Queen could see to that? And Miss Nightingale would like the Queen to get the military cemeteries near the hospital at Scutari brought under British control. Queen Victoria moved swiftly to grant Miss Nightingale both of these urgent requests.

The sick and dying men in Miss Nightingale's wards knew that superior and powerful as she was they could always rely on receiving from her a gentle and compassionate word:

> 'I believe', wrote one of the civilian doctors who was
> working in the Scutari Hospital, 'that there was never a
> severe case of any kind that escaped her notice, and
> sometimes it was wonderful to see her at the bedside of a
> patient who had been admitted perhaps an hour before,
> and of whose arrival one would hardly have supposed she
> could be already cognisant'.[19]

Her nurses were inspired by her manner to the men. 'It was so
tender and kind',[20] wrote one of them. Her patients came
near to worshipping her. 'What a comfort it was to see her
pass, even', wrote one soldier. 'She would speak to one, and
nod and smile to as many more; but she could not do it all you
know. We lay there by hundreds; but we could kiss her
shadow as it fell and lay our heads on the pillow again
content'.[21]

Miss Nightingale could have returned to Britain, after the
emergency in the Crimea was over, in the rôle of a national
heroine, with men-of-war provided by the Government to
take her home in state, battalions of guardsmen to escort her
to and from the men-of-war, and grand processions mounted
specially, once she was safely back on English soil, to solve
her remaining personal travelling difficulties. But Miss
Nightingale preferred to move quietly back towards Britain
under her own steam. She travelled incognito, spending just
one night in Paris with a friend of her family's, and crossing
the Channel, after that, in as unmarked a fashion as any
ordinary twentieth-century holiday tourist. Totally exhausted by the physical and mental agonies she had suffered
during the previous two years, Florence Nightingale spent a
few hours in London: she crept off quietly to the Convent of
the Bermondsey Nuns and calmed herself there, with the
Reverend Mother, in prayers and meditation. Later in the
same day, Miss Nightingale took a train north – she was still
travelling strictly incognito – and, somehow, she managed to

get herself to the entrance of the long drive of her family's northernmost home, Lea Hurst. Mrs Watson, the house-keeper, happened to be sitting in her room in the front of the house a few minutes later and, happening to look out of her window, she saw the nation's heroine walking, unannounced, towards the front door. Mrs Watson screamed – in the best traditions of Victorian melodrama – and then rushed out of the house to greet the uncrowned Queen of Scutari.

During the next few months Florence Nightingale ought to have been content, one would have thought, to rest. Any normal woman, if she had survived what Miss Nightingale had gone through, would have allowed herself to be restored by careful nursing to her former states of physical and mental health. But Florence Nightingale was far from being a normal person. She was a fanatic, who was determined to carry on intensively the extraordinary work she had been doing in the Crimea – work that had been so successful that the general public had practically ceased to think of British private soldiers as ignorant brutes and of the women who nursed them as drunken whores. Both – soldiers and nurses – had been raised immeasurably in status by Miss Nightingale's efforts and she had not the slightest intention of allowing them to sink again to their former levels of degradation.

To help her in her campaign, Florence Nightingale had certain unprecedented advantages. First, she managed to get the Queen and the Prince Consort wholeheartedly to support her. Invited by the Royal Physician, Sir James Clark, to stay at his Scottish home, Birk Hall, which was near Balmoral, so that she could meet the Royal couple, Miss Nightingale quickly earned the respect and even the affection of the Sovereign and her Consort. 'She put before us all the defects of our present military hospital system, and the reforms that are needed', recorded the Queen after Miss Nightingale's first interview with her. 'We are much pleased with her; she is extremely modest'.[22] A few days later the Queen drove over to Birk Hall and the ladies had 'tea and a great talk'.[23] Miss

Nightingale knew exactly what she wanted – before the complete reorganisation of the army medical services could be achieved, she saw clearly, a Royal commission would have to be appointed – but she and the Queen would have to deal, first, with Lord Panmure, who had taken Sidney Herbert's place as Minister of War, and who was immensely skilled in the difficult art of avoiding trouble. The best way of doing this, Lord Panmure had found, was to take no positive action of any kind unless this became absolutely inevitable. The Queen's resolution and Miss Nightingale's charming modesty were too much for Lord Panmure and he agreed, albeit unwillingly, that the Royal Commission that Miss Nightingale wanted so urgently should be set up.

To start her great work of reform moving was one thing; to keep it in motion was quite another, when the Minister of War was dilatory, the Permanent Under Secretary at the War Office, Sir Benjamin Hawes, was implacably opposed to the very idea of change, and a host of other and lesser people were ready to do everything they could to thwart Miss Nightingale in the achievement of her aims. Though she was temperamentally averse to seeking personal publicity of any kind, Miss Nightingale was at length driven to making use of the second of her incomparable advantages – the immense admiration with which she was regarded by the vast majority of Queen Victoria's subjects. 'Three months from this day I publish my experiences of the Crimean campaign, and my suggestions for improvement', she wrote threateningly in the late winter of 1856–7, 'unless there has been a fair and tangible pledge by that time for reform'.[24] Her threats were heard, and acted upon.

The mortal illness of Sidney Herbert who, if he had remained in good health, would have made an incomparable Chairman of Miss Nightingale's Royal Commission, was a serious setback that not even Miss Nightingale, with all her resolution and tenacity, could overcome. She fought on indomitably, however, as Sidney Herbert's strength failed, compiling in the process a monumental work which was nearly a thousand pages long and was plentifully supplied with authoritative statistics. In this work, which she called *Notes on Matters affecting the Health, Efficiency and Hospital Administration of the British Army*, Miss Nightingale was able to show unanswerably that the medical authorities of the Army of the past few decades had been, quite literally, killers. For every man who had fallen in battle or who had died of wounds in the Crimean War, she contended, seven had died from diseases which could with proper care have been prevented. In peacetime too, she demonstrated, the medical authorities of the Army had been culpable. Soldiers, she stressed, were young, strong and vigorous men, but their rate of mortality was double, and often more than double, the rate of mortality of the population as a whole – and that was taking into account the old and senile, the newly born, and the women who were exposed to the grave risks of childbirth. In the parish of St Pancras – and this was only one of several chilling instances she gave – the general rate of mortality was 2·2 per thousand; in the Life Guards' barracks, which stood in that parish, the rate was 10·4 per thousand. 'Fifteen hundred good soldiers are as certainly killed by these neglects yearly as if they were drawn up on Salisbury Plain and shot', she alleged. She added scathingly 'Our soldiers enlist to death in the barracks'.[25]

While she was apparently wholly engrossed with the affairs of the Army, Miss Nightingale was dealing with several other problems that urgently needed her attention. She was passionately interested in the design of hospitals and travelled long distances, while she was still in a very low state of health, to inspect such institutions. Before long, she was recognised as the country's leading expert on the subject, and her advice was so often sought that she had to spend several hours practically every day, dealing with the correspondence that poured in on her from many different parts of the world.

In 1859 the Governors of the ancient St Thomas's Hospital in London were offered a large sum of money by the Directors of the South-Eastern Railway Company for part of their land. It was almost inevitable that Miss Nightingale should be consulted by the hospital's Resident Medical Officer. Did Miss Nightingale recommend that the land that the railway company required should be sold and that the hospital should be partially rebuilt on what remained of its traditional site? Or did she think that the land in Southwark should be given up altogether, and that the entire hospital should be rebuilt on more modern lines, possibly in another and healthier part of London? After carrying out much detailed research, Miss Nightingale came down emphatically in favour of the second alternative and wrote to the Prince Consort, who was a Governor of the hospital, to tell him so. Her opinion was so highly regarded that all debate on the subject was virtually at an end. By 1871, a new St Thomas's, built on the 'pavilion' plan especially favoured by Miss Nightingale, had been put up on the fine Thames-side site in Lambeth where the recently-enlarged hospital stands to this day.

While she was first being drawn, in an advisory capacity, into the affairs of St Thomas's Hospital, Miss Nightingale had on her mind one of the greatest of all her schemes – the creation of a proper training school for female nurses. There was money available to pay for such a school – the 'Nightingale Fund', raised by public subscription shortly after the end of the Crimean War as a tribute to her great achievements, would, alone, provide some £45,000 – and, she had found earlier at St Thomas's a remarkable woman named Mrs Wardroper who was Matron of the hospital and who, Miss Nightingale declared in a letter to Sidney Herbert, was the only Matron 'of any existing Hospital' that she would recommend to form a School of Instruction for Nurses. It would not be the *best conceivable* way of beginning, added Miss Nightingale with a tinge of regret, for it would be beginning in a very humble way. But it did seem to her to be the best way possible under the circumstances.

Shortly after that, Miss Nightingale and Mrs Wardroper embarked on Miss Nightingale's great project, though the

Matron warned Miss Nightingale that the scheme might receive from the more conservative doctors on the hospital's staff some 'rather harsh criticism'. Undeterred, Miss Nightingale produced and had published a short book which she named *Notes on Nursing: What it is, and what it is not*. The book was full of good sense and practical suggestions, emphasising the importance of hygiene which, the authoress specified, involved the provision of plenty of fresh air, cleanliness, pure water, satisfactory drainage and plenty of light. Miss Nightingale stressed, too, the nurse's need to consider the feelings of her patient – the sick being, in Miss Nightingale's view, so much more sensitive and more easily upset than those in perfect health. 'I shall never forget the rapture of fever patients over a bunch of bright-coloured flowers', she wrote. Then, recalling her own sufferings from fever at Scutari, she added 'I remember in my own case a nosegay of wild flowers being sent me, and from that moment recovery became more rapid'. The book was an immediate success, fifteen thousand copies being sold within four weeks of its first appearance. It was translated, then, into several foreign languages as well as being published in America. 'There is not one word in it written for the sake of writing but only forced out of me by much experience of human suffering' was Miss Nightingale's own verdict on her small but authoritative treatise.[26]

The Nightingale Training School for Nurses opened at St Thomas's Hospital just a few months after the publication of *Notes on Nursing*. Fifteen probationers, selected only after the most rigorous investigation into their pasts and potentialities, were enrolled; given separate bedrooms and the use of a communal sitting room; fitted out with neat brown uniforms with white caps and aprons; granted £10 each to cover the personal expenses they might incur while they were being trained; and promised cash bonuses, calculated according to their proficiency, when they had completed their courses. They were required to attend daily lectures given by the medical staff and the sisters of the hospital; to take notes from those lectures; to be ready to submit their notebooks, at any time, for inspection by Mrs Wardroper or by Miss Nightingale, and to keep personal diaries (which were also liable to be scanned, at a moment's notice, by Miss Nightingale's eagle eye). A number of the senior members of the surgical and medical staff of the hospital grumbled, as Mrs Wardroper had predicted that they would, at the unprecedented amount of fuss that was being made over the young women. Nurses, in their disgruntled view, were little more than housemaids and needed to be taught only how to scrub and how to make poultices. But the Matron and Miss Nightingale pressed on with their great enterprise, chiding gently a probationer whose moral character was said to be 'unexceptionable' but who seemed to be unable to prevent herself from 'using her eyes unpleasantly'. They threatened with instant dismissal any probationer who might be tempted to flirt.

Soon a flood of letters was arriving at the school at St Thomas's from those who wished to engage the Nightingale probationers as soon as their periods of training had been satisfactorily completed. Thirteen out of the fifteen young women were judged to have 'qualified', were placed officially on a 'register', and left to take up permanent employment in hospitals and infirmaries where their unimpeachable conduct and exceptional abilities were to advertise further the excellence of the Nightingale School. The fame of the school spread abroad, most conspicuously perhaps in Prussia, where, largely as a result of Miss Nightingale's personal friendship with Queen Victoria's daughter the Crown Princess, the Victoria School of Nurses was set up on the St Thomas's lines, and in America, where Clare Barton, founder of the American Red Cross, helped to set the highest possible standards for the rapidly developing nursing profession.

While Miss Nightingale was devoting so much energy to the proper training of nurses, other people in Britain, inspired by her example, were founding and fitting out 'cottage hospitals' that would serve, in the new enlightened age, rural areas and the smaller country towns.

The first 'cottage hospital' is believed to have been founded by a Doctor Albert Napper at Cranleigh, in Surrey, in 1859. He called it a 'village hospital', but in 1867 a Doctor E. J. Waring, author of several books and pamphlets on the subject, suggested that the name 'cottage hospital' would define more satisfactorily the real nature of the establishment. 'The cottage element should never be lost sight of', he prescribed. 'The building should in all cases be a cottage – a model cottage, if circumstances permit – with all the advantages of efficient drainage, good ventilation, and a cheerful exterior, but still essentially a cottage in character and pretension'.[27]

By 1865, there were eighteen cottage hospitals in various parts of the country. By 1880, there were nearly two hundred, and there were only five counties in the whole of England which could not boast of at least one.

Medical and surgical care in the cottage hospitals would normally be provided by the local General Practitioners. These country doctors would find that their professional status would be raised considerably in the eyes of their patients and potential patients by their association with the tiny local 'infirmary'. And they could carry out, in their local cottage hospitals, much more serious operations than they could have attempted in their own or their patients' homes.

For a few years after the development of anaesthetics, the cottage hospitals of Britain – relatively free from the gross infections that seethed through the crowded wards of the larger city hospitals – offered surgical patients the best possible chance of survival. It was only after the antiseptic methods of Sir Joseph Lister and the hygienic techniques of Miss Nightingale became generally accepted that the larger hospitals also managed to achieve a lower rate of mortality.

In her later life, Miss Nightingale became a permanent invalid and something of a recluse – no one, even a Monarch, could be admitted to her presence without a previous appointment – but she did not cease to take the closest possible interest in the probationers who were joining, passing through, or leaving 'her' school, and she kept in touch with many of her favourite ex-students through the rest of their professional careers. She went to extraordinary pains to make each and every one of 'her' nurses feel extra-important. When a Miss Torrance was made Matron of the Highgate Hospital, for instance, Miss Nightingale wrote more than one hundred letters to her in her first year of office, and had to read about the same number of replies. 'I have never been used to influence people except by leading in WORK', she grumbled to a family friend, 'and to have to influence them by talking and writing is hard. A more dreadful thing than being cut short by death is being cut short by life in a paralysed state'.[28] When any of 'her' nurses went to a new post, Miss Nightingale would send flowers to make her immediately feel at home. Miss Nightingale's nurses, in consequence, almost without exception worshipped her. 'That I have seen Miss Nightingale will be one of the white milestones on my road',[29] declared one of them a little unctuously. But this young woman's high opinion of Miss Nightingale was perhaps justified, for in a little over thirty years Miss Nightingale had managed, in her own words, to raise nursing 'from the sink'. By the end of the nineteenth century it had become, due almost entirely to her unceasing efforts, one of the most worthwhile and admired of all human activities.

In June 1907, members of an International Conference of Red Cross Societies, meeting in London, sent a message to 'Miss Florence Nightingale, the pioneer of the first Red Cross movement, whose heroic efforts on behalf of suffering humanity will be recognised and admired by all ages as long as the world shall last'.[30] Three years later (it was the Jubilee of the foundation of the Nightingale Training School at St Thomas's Hospital) a meeting was held in the Carnegie Hall in New York at which the Public Orator spoke with great feeling of the great record and of the noble life of Miss Florence Nightingale. There were already, he said, more than one thousand training schools for nurses in the United States alone. But Miss Nightingale was by that time too old and ill to appreciate anything that was being said about her. She died peacefully in her sleep, on 13 August 1910, one of the most eminent of all Eminent Victorians.

# 9

# The Start of Modern Orthopaedics

*. . . Thou shalt make me hear of joy and gladness: that*
*the bones which thou hast broken may rejoice . . .*

Psalm 49

What to do with human bodies in which the bones were broken or distorted? That question had been asked, and not properly answered, since the days of the psalmist, and probably for very much longer than that.

In the early eighteenth century William Cheselden, principal surgeon at St Thomas's Hospital, London, was an enthusiastic advocate of egg-white bandages for the treatment of fractures and for the correction of club feet, and egg-white remained a popular bonding agent for many decades. In Arabia, during the same period, plaster was being used. Mr Eton, the British consul in Bassora, wrote in 1798:

> I saw in the Eastern parts of the Empire a method of setting bones practised which appears to be worthy of the attention of surgeons in Europe. It is by enclosing the broken limb, after the bones are put in their places, in a case of plaster of Paris (gypsum) which takes exactly the form of the limb, without any pressure, and in a few minutes the mass is solid and strong. There is nothing in gypsum injurious, if it be free from lime.[1]

In India, similar methods were used. Sir George Ballingall wrote in *Outline of Military Surgery*, in 1852:

> The practice of enveloping fractured limbs in splints and bandages, without undoing them, for weeks together, is

117

akin to that followed by the natives of India of enclosing fractured limbs in moulds of clay. Of the successful results of this practice I remember a remarkable instance in the case of a little boy who was brought into my tent one morning, having been run over by a waggon on the line of march, and having sustained a severe compound fracture of the leg. I was preparing to amputate this boy's limb when the parents came in and carried him away to a potter in an adjoining village, who enveloped the leg in clay, and I believe finally cured the patient.

In Europe, a surgeon named Hubenthal is said to have used plaster of Paris in 1816. He mixed the plaster with torn up blotting paper. Twelve years after that, Kluge and Koyle introduced a plaster box to the Charité Hospital in Berlin. Their method was to lay the injured limb in a wooden box into which plaster was poured. Gentin, who was the senior Medical Officer of the Belgian Army, recommended the use of starch bandages in 1834 in an attempt to keep walking those of his patients who had fractures of the leg. Another Army surgeon – Mathysen, of the Dutch Army – introduced plaster bandages in 1852. It was Hugh Owen Thomas, though, who may be fairly called the Founding Father of modern orthopaedics.

Hugh Owen Thomas came from a family who lived in a remote part of the island of Anglesey. For four generations – ever since two young boys had been rescued from a shipwreck and adopted by the family – the Thomas menfolk had been practising as 'meddygon esgyrn', or bone setters, though their main source of income had been their farms.

At last, in the early nineteenth century, one of the bone-setting Thomases – Evan – felt himself drawn to the rapidly growing seaport town of Liverpool. There he acquired a considerable reputation as a skilful manipulator. The place of an anaesthetic during Evan Thomas's 'operations' was taken by a music box, worked by his man, which was intended to distract the patient's attention and, possibly, to drown his groans during the most painful parts of the proceedings.

Hugh Owen, the first child of Evan Thomas, was born in Anglesey on 23 August 1834 while his mother was visiting her parents there. After his school years, the young Hugh Owen was apprenticed to an uncle of his who was a doctor at St Asaph. In 1854, when he was just 21, he became a medical student at Edinburgh. After three years there, he spent a year at University College Hospital, London. Then he spent a short time in Paris, studying the methods of the French surgeons. In 1858, he returned to Liverpool so that he could be an assistant in his father's practice. The partnership did not last, though – probably because the father, who was not a professionally qualified man, could not or would not accept his son's 'new-fangled' ideas. In addition, the orthodox medical practitioners of the town were becoming increasingly critical of Evan, whom they considered an untrained and possibly dangerous outsider. Evan, for his part, defended his methods with an abrupt 'I never "suppose". If I am in doubt I never undertake a case'.[2]

Unable to work in harmony with his father and his brother, Hugh Owen Thomas, in 1859, set up in practice on his own. Immediately, he was inundated with patients from the teeming dockside tenements and from the accident-prone seafaring community.

During more than thirty years of intensive work after that, Hugh Owen Thomas only allowed himself to be away from home for some six nights. At six o'clock every morning he would set off on his rounds, using for transport a dog-cart which he had designed himself and had had made, on his own premises, by his own workmen. He would see between thirty and forty patients in a single morning, dressing their wounds, prescribing and dispensing medicines for them and, where necessary, treating their fractures and reducing their dislocations, often without expecting any financial reward. On Sunday mornings, instead of allowing himself a rest, he would hold a 'free clinic' when as many as two hundred impoverished patients would gather at his consulting rooms.

Working almost without ceasing in this way, Hugh Owen Thomas managed to develop, on his own initiative, the modern treatment of fractures. He was completely opposed to the growing practice of immobilising limbs with plaster since this, in his view, 'did not allow frequent inspection, was much labour at first, and little afterwards, and provided no opportunity for the display of skill'.[3] He despised the rudimentary wooden splints that were used by most practitioners of the time for supporting limbs with broken bones – if, indeed, those limbs were supported at all. He believed passionately that an injured limb should be given a complete rest. At the same time he believed, equally emphatically, that a patient should be kept as far as possible active and in full employment. 'A man who understands my principles will do better with a bandage and a broomstick than another can do with an instrument-maker's arsenal', he used to claim.[4]

The premises on which, and from which, Hugh Owen Thomas worked were so well equipped that he had to call in no aid from outside. Needing relatively sophisticated splints of every size, that would suit any type of fracture that might occur, or any deformity that might need treatment, he decided to use, principally, iron for strength and rigidity and leather for comfortable padding. He was a capable mechanic himself but, to assist him, he decided to employ a full-time blacksmith, who worked in Thomas's own smithy; a saddler, who finished off the splints; and other assistants who made adhesive plasters and bandages of all kinds and prepared the dressings he needed. On Hugh Owen Thomas's home-made splints, many of our most necessary modern orthopaedic appliances are based.

There is no doubt that Hugh Owen Thomas was years ahead of his time, and the results of his treatment of fractures and of tuberculous arthritis seemed, to the professional observers who attended his clinics, little short of miraculous. A Doctor John Ridlon, of Chicago, who had read Thomas's book *Hip, Knee and Ankle*, travelled more than three thousand miles to watch the great Liverpool medical man at work. Ridlon reported:

I will now recall some of the cases I saw . . . A man with a fractured patella is brought in by his fellow workmen. A leg splint is brought down from the loft, the distal end cut off, the ring snugly fitted by bending the side rods at their attachment to it, the lower ends again cut off to desired length and their ends bent to right angles and fitted into a hole in the heel of the shoe that had been drilled through it, two pads of sheet-iron padded on one side with felt were bent by hand to troughs to fit the front of the thigh and the shin, and these fastened by bandage half-hitched around the side rods, and passing obliquely so that the upper one crowded the upper fragment of the patella downwards and the lower one upwards, with the joint fully straight. The man is told that he can return to work and walks away.[5]

It is ironic that on one of the few occasions Hugh Owen Thomas left his practice, in the 1870s, he went to offer the use of the Thomas Splint to the French Army. His offer was refused. Nearly half a century later, Thomas's nephew Robert Jones was to record:

The Great War afforded the most convincing proof of the mishandling of complicated, and even of simple, fractures. Fractures of the femur serve as a notable example. The splint with which we are all so familiar, invented by Thomas, was barely known, and yet it was the type of splint which ultimately saved the situation. In 1916 the mortality from these fractures amounted to 80 per cent, a large proportion of the deaths occuring on their way to or at the Casualty Clearing Stations. Later, when the Thomas Splint was applied almost exclusively, and as near to the firing line as possible, the mortality in 1918 was reduced to 20 per cent.[6]

Hugh Owen Thomas died in 1891, quite worn out by his continuous exertions.

*I 0*

# Blood and Blood Transfusions

*. . . 'Let there be light!' said God, and there was light!*
*'Let there be blood!' says man, and there's a sea . . .*

LORD BYRON (1788–1824), *Don Juan*

From the start of history, the blood has been regarded as one of the most important ingredients of animal economy, no doubt because it has always been obvious that loss of blood is followed by loss of life as inevitably as spring follows winter. So blood came to be invested with many mysterious properties, and in the days of the Roman Empire it was believed that the weak could increase their strength by bathing in, or drinking, the blood of the strong. The blood of bulls or of gladiators killed in the arena was particularly valued as a tonic beverage.[1]

In 1657, Sir Christopher Wren carried out a 'Noble Anatomical Experiment of injecting Liquors into the Veins of Animals', and his research was described in some detail by Robert Boyle in his *Usefulnesse of Experimental Philosophy* published in 1663. In May 1665, the distinguished members of the British Royal Society entered in their journal book:

> It was ordered that the experiment of injecting the blood of one dog into another be tried at the next meeting: upon which occasion Dr Croune suggested that a common pipe might be used for both, in order to have thereby the blood of one dog sucked out by the other.

Towards the end of February 1666, Richard Lower carried out an experiment of paramount importance in the history of blood transfusion when he transferred blood directly from the artery of one dog to the vein of another. The members of the Royal Society, encouraged by this, played with the idea of transfusing blood into a human being. In his Diary, later that year, Samuel Pepys reported:

> At the meeting at Gresham College tonight . . . There was a pretty experiment of the blood of one dogg let out, till he died, into the body of another on one side while all his own run out on the other side. The first upon the place, and the other very well, and likely to do well. This did give occasion to many pretty wishes, as of the blood of a Quaker to be let into an Archbishop, and such like; but, as Dr Croune says, may, if it takes, be of mighty use to man's health, for the amending of bad blood by borrowing from a better body . . .

In November 1667, Pepys reported that a 'poor and debauched man', a failed scholar from Cambridge, had had the blood of a sheep let into his body. In Paris, shortly before this, Jean Denys, Professor of Philosophy and Mathematics and physician to Louis XIV, had claimed that he had successfully carried out an animal-to-man transfusion, but Denys's self-satisfaction was not to last, for in the following year one of his patients died after the third of a series of transfusions and the widow instituted proceedings against him. The case caused much excitement, which mounted when the widow was accused of poisoning her husband. After the case, from which Denys emerged with some discredit, orders were given that in future no blood transfusion of any kind might be carried out without the permission of a member of the Faculty of Medicine of Paris. As the members of the Faculty were bitterly opposed to the whole idea, the necessary permission was never granted and the practice of transfusion, in France, was brought speedily to an end. In England, a few more experiments were carried out with animals. Here, too, the idea was allowed to lapse for more than a century.

It is not really surprising that so many of the earliest

attempts to transfuse blood were to prove dangerous, for no one was sufficiently knowledgeable to appreciate that animal blood, be it of dog, lamb or calf, contains proteins that are totally incompatible with those found in human blood. The first intimation that this might be the case did not come until the second and third decades of the nineteenth century when the physician and obstetrician James Blundell (born 1790) was driven by his helplessness in the face of the severe haemorrhages that were liable to follow childbirth to experiment with transfusion. Blundell, later, observed:

> For the original operation the presence of some animal in the bed-chamber was necessary; what then was to be done in an emergency? A dog, it is true, might have come when you whistled, but the animal is small; a calf or a sheep might, to some, have appeared fitter for the purpose; but then it could not run upstairs. In this condition of it, the operation, little more than a name, was great in its danger, but of small advantage in those very cases of sudden bleeding in which it seems most required.[2]

Doctor Blundell was saved from making the same basic mistakes as his predecessors by a colleague, Doctor Leacock of Barbados, who suggested that the blood of animals might not be beneficial and might even be positively harmful to human beings. Realising that the blood of any one species might not be suitable for another species, Doctor Blundell carried out a lengthy series of experiments on dogs. He proved, first, that a dog which had been bled almost to the point of death could be revived and restored fully to health if it were given the blood of another dog. Next he showed that if a dog that had been bled was given the blood of a sheep, it would invariably die, even though it appeared, at the start, to make a partial recovery. From these researches came the doctrine on which all modern blood transfusion procedure is based.

On 22 December 1818, Doctor Blundell gave the members of the Medico-Chirurgical Society in London an account of an operation in which he had given an incurably ill patient from twelve to fourteen ounces of blood, drawn from several human donors by means of a syringe. The patient survived for fifty-six hours after the operation, and this encouraged Doctor Blundell to perform further transfusions when suitable opportunities occurred. An account of a successful transfusion carried out by Doctor Blundell is given in *The Lancet* (1829), and it seems probable that he did others, using a rudimentary funnel-and-pump instrument that he called an 'impellor'. Later, he devised another instrument, the 'gravitator', in which, as its name implies, the force of gravity is used for pushing the blood into the vein of the patient. In the course of his work, Blundell managed to prove conclusively that the introduction of a few air bubbles into a patient's circulation was relatively harmless, and not, as had been previously believed, apt to be fatal.

Many of the technical difficulties which had faced those experimenting with blood transfusion were removed after 1853 by the invention of the hypodermic syringe, with its hollow pointed needle. Credit for the evolution of this universally useful appliance is usually given to Doctor Alexander Wood (born 1817), who was appointed Secretary of the Royal College of Physicians of Edinburgh in 1850. For some time, Doctor Wood had been experimenting with a hollow needle for the administration of drugs. Eventually, he felt confident enough to publish in *The Edinburgh Medical and Surgical Review* a short paper – 'A New Method of treating Neuralgia by the direct application of Opiates to the Painful Points' – in which he showed that the method was not necessarily limited to the administration of opiates. At about the same time, Charles Gabriel Pravaz of Lyon was making a similar syringe which quickly came into use in many surgeries under the name of 'The Pravaz Syringe'.

In 1863, Doctor J.H. Aveling, an obstetrician, was experimenting with a simple but effective piece of apparatus which consisted, principally, of two silver tubes to enter the emittent and recipient blood vessels, two stop-cocks, and a length of indiarubber tube to carry the blood between the two parties. There was a small bulb in the middle of this tube. If this bulb were pressed between the thumb and the forefinger, it would act as an auxiliary heart. For more than eight years the doctor carried this device in his pocket to every confinement he attended. At last, in 1872, he found an opportunity to use it when he was called to a lady, aged twenty-one, who was *in extremis* from post-partum haemorrhage. Quickly, Doctor Aveling managed to give her sixty drachms of blood, which he obtained from her coachman. The lady soon recovered sufficiently to be able to remark that she was dying, though, Doctor Aveling observed, 'the mental improvement was not as marked and rapid as I anticipated, but this was, perhaps, due to the quantity of brandy she had taken'. The coachman, he was pleased to record, was not only collected and cheerful, but able to make several useful suggestions during the process of transfusion.

Once the value of the transfusion of human blood as a life-saving measure had been established, urgent research had to be carried out into the main technical difficulty – the tendency of the blood to clot and, in doing so, to block the tubes and other contrivances in the process. One of the first men to make any progress in this direction was Braxton Hicks, an obstetrician of Guy's Hospital, who was advised to use phosphate of sodium as an anticoagulant. In 1883–4 he performed four transfusions using blood mixed with one-fourth its volume of a solution of sodium phosphate. No clotting occurred. All four patients died, however – a result in which the poisonous properties of sodium phosphate may have played some part.

In 1873, at St Bartholomew's Hospital, Sir Thomas Smith successfully gave blood from which the clot had been removed ('defibrinated' blood) to an infant suffering from haemorrhage of the newly born. The use of defibrinated blood for transfusions then became fairly general, but the removal of the clot, usually by means of a hair-sieve, was a slow and laborious process, and as it also removed much of the protein of the blood and many of the cells it radically reduced the blood's value to the recipient.

Between 1891 and the outbreak of the First World War, several investigators were experimenting with possible anticoagulants – among the many substances tried and discarded being hirudin, peptone and sodium citrate. At last, in 1914, L. Agote, working in Buenos Aires, and Richard Lewisohn, in New York, almost simultaneously established that sodium citrate would indeed be both effective and safe, so long as the total amount of citrate administered did not exceed five grams. By 1917 the citrate method was being widely used in casualty clearing stations and military hospitals in France.

Meanwhile, another advance of fundamental importance had been made. In 1907, the four blood groups known as O, A, B and AB had been identified by J. Jansky, working at the Sbornik Klinicky in Prague, and his discoveries were confirmed in 1910 by W.L. Moss of the Johns Hopkins Hospital, Baltimore. It was possible, after that, to eliminate most of the fatalities that could result from the use of incompatible blood. The tests could be carried out and the blood groups of both donor and recipient could be established with reasonable accuracy in a few minutes, too, so that the safeguard could be used even in an emergency. Before long, methods of blood transfusion had been devised that united the four cardinal virtues of certainty, efficiency, safety and simplicity. In the late 1930s it came into extensive and general use.

## II

# Spas and Watering-Places during the Nineteenth Century

*. . . Water, water everywhere . . .*

SAMUEL TAYLOR COLERIDGE (1772–1834)
*The Rime of the Ancient Mariner*

'One would think the English were ducks; they are for ever waddling to the waters', wrote Horace Walpole in 1790, with an unmistakable air of condescension. In the previous year, King George III had set the seal of royal approval on the newly fashionable activity of sea-bathing by entering the waves off Weymouth.

During the reigns of King George I and George II, Bath, with its thermal springs, had been a favourite out-of-town meeting place of the highly fashionable. It was King George III's eldest son, George, Prince of Wales, who preferred the little Sussex village of Brighthelmstone, now Brighton, and his friends and cronies, disliking the middle-class people who were daring, by that time, to go to Bath, were only too ready to join him there.

By the last years of the eighteenth century, a steadily increasing number of people, following the royal lead, were being persuaded that good health could be regained as effectively by immersion in sea water as by immersion in the water of an inland spa. Poor Robert Burns, suffering in 1796 from acute rheumatism and prolonged lowering of the spirits, was ordered by his medical advisers to wade each day into the cold grey waters of the Solway until those waters came up to his armpits. 'It would be an injustice to deny that it [sea bathing] has eased my pains', Burns wrote courageously to Mrs Burns, 'and I think has strengthened me; but my appetite is still extremely bad'.[1] Dragging his aching limbs out of the icy Atlantic water, the tortured poet would dry himself with the utmost difficulty and would then lower a carefully measured glass of reinvigorating port wine. The treatment did Burns little good, however, for within a few months he was dead. But in spite of several similar reverses, the advocates of sea-bathing pressed on.

The increasing popularity of Brighton as a meeting place for the rich and influential during the early years of the nineteenth century did not noticeably lessen the drawing power of the established inland watering places. Cheltenham, where King George III had stayed, prospered sufficiently, in fact, to incur the disapproval of William Cobbett, author of *Rural Rides*, who, in 1821, described the town as 'a nasty ill-looking place, half clown and half-cockney', adding, when he returned there reluctantly in 1826, that it was 'a place to which East India plunderers, West India floggers, English tax-gorgers, together with gluttonous drinkers and debauchees of all descriptions, female as well as male, resort, at the suggestion of silently laughing quacks, in the hope of getting rid of the bodily consequences of their manifold sins and iniquities'. When he entered a place like Cheltenham, he went on, he always felt disposed to squeeze up his nose with his fingers:

> To places like this come all that is knavish and all that is base; gamesters, pickpockets and harlots; young wife-hunters in search of rich and ugly old women and young husband-hunters in search of rich and wrinkled or half-rotten men, the former resolutely bent, be the means what they may, to give the latter heirs to their lands and tenements.

Cobbett claimed, mistakenly, that this 'nasty stupid spot' was already in decline and would be entirely deserted within a year or so. On principle, he refused to spend a single penny in the place. In spite of Cobbett's radical forecasts, Cheltenham remained, until well after the end of the nineteenth century, one of Britain's most respected spas.

Leamington, in Warwickshire, had been only a rough encampment of crude huts before William Abbotts, in 1786, had found a vigorous mineral spring on his own land there and had decided to exploit it. Then further springs giving chalybeate, saline, and sulphurous waters were discovered in the immediate neighbourhood, and elegant bath-houses, designed in the fashionable classical style, were put up for the convenience of those who might be attracted to Leamington for a 'cure'. This word was used, at the time, to describe a course of treatment rather than the successful outcome of such a course. Visited by the Prince Regent and by the Princess Victoria and her mother the Duchess of Kent, the handsome new town that had been laid out around the classical bath-houses was allowed, in the year after the accession of Victoria as Queen, to call itself a 'Royal Spa'. From that moment on, the proprietors of the expensive hotels that had sprung up in the town spoke about Leamington as if the place were as important as Carlsbad and Marienbad and the other well-known Continental spas. An expert on those spas – Doctor Augustus Bozzi Granville, who had visited all the best-known German watering places and had written in glowing terms about most of them – was persuaded, in the cause of fairness, to undertake a similar tour of inspection in the British Isles. After visiting the Royal Leamington Spa, Doctor Granville reported that there were no 'ambiguous characters' there – such people could not possibly afford to visit Leamington, he suggested. But the absence of all undesirable characters was offset, he said, by the inadequacy of the saline spring, the water from which was not much better than ordinary sea water, if as good. However, Leamington Spa survived Doctor Granville's strictures as successfully as Cheltenham had survived those of William Cobbett.

Harrogate's special but unusually nasty-smelling waters,

said to have been discovered by William Slingsby, a local landowner, as far back as 1571, were attracting a small number of faithful patrons by the end of the eighteenth century, but as the tiny village had too little accommodation most of these had to stay in nearby Knaresborough. By the end of the Napoleonic wars, the town had grown considerably in size and it had acquired a permanent theatre and a racecourse. As further wells were discovered after that, in or near the town, there was no shortage of private speculators ready to build, equip and provide the staff for pump rooms and mineral baths; to lay out parks and gardens; and to provide all the other attractive features of a fashionable spa. In the second half of the nineteenth century the municipal authorities undertook further to expand Harrogate, and by the end of Queen Victoria's reign the Yorkshire spa, with more than forty different types of mineral bath on offer, was able to compete with any of the more renowned Continental watering places. Early in the present century, the Harrogate authorities even provided brine baths containing water moved specially by rail from the North Sea.

Long before King George III went into the sea off Weymouth, the members of mixed bathing parties had been going into the waves off the beach at Scarborough, and there were two changing rooms, one for each sex, at the Yorkshire resort years before any such amenities were provided for the sea bathers at Brighthelmstone. With the arrival of the railway, Scarborough – 'The Queen of the Northern Watering Places', as the resort was called in many advertisements – it could easily have become a run-of-the-mill holiday centre, overrun in good weather by crowds of excursionists and day trippers. But the local authorities were determined that their town should cater only for the wealthy and refined, and Scarborough managed to retain its anachronistic 'select Regency spa' atmosphere right up to the First World War.

While the growth of some spa towns was encouraged, during the nineteenth century, by the arrival of railways, the popularity of others was increased dramatically by a fashionable interest in 'hydropathy'. The advantages of this cold water therapy had been advocated as far back as 1697, when Sir John Floyer, a physician of Lichfield, Staffordshire, published a treatise to be called *The Ancient Psychrolusia*. In this, Sir John drew his readers' attention to the people of certain semi-civilised nations such as the Tartars, the Muscovites, the Irish and the Scottish, who, he wrote, were in the habit of toughening themselves and their offspring by the act of immersion in very cold water. Many of Sir John's patients allowed themselves to be dipped in icy water, usually after they had been bled or purged and told not to eat before the treatment. Ten years later, a Doctor Browne of London and Bath, who knew and admired Sir John's teachings, published *An Account of the Wonderful Cures Performed by the Cold Baths*.[2] Among the patients who, he said, had been cured by cold water therapy was Sir Henry Blount, of Tittenhanger, Hertfordshire, who had 'found the greatest relief by the constant use of cold water poured into his shoes several times a day, though in the hardest frost of winter'. Also quoted was a goldsmith of Lombard Street who had had holes cut in the soles of his boots so that the healing damp might be admitted. All through the eighteenth century, after that, advocates of 'wetting and sweating' were to be heard claiming that with these two elementary treatments and without the use of drugs they could cure an extraordinary range of illnesses and could repair, too, most of the ravages caused by human frailty.[3]

It was a farmer's son called Vincent Priessnitz, however, who first raised hydropathy to the status of an international cult.

Priessnitz was born in 1799. He operated, in the first instance, in and near the little town of Gräfenberg, which was set at an altitude of two thousand feet in the mountains of Silesia. The town is now in Czechoslovakia, and is known as 'Jesenik'. The Gräfenberg waters had no unusual chemical characteristics, so no attempt was ever made to advertise

Gräfenberg as a spa. Nor were any grand or pretentious buildings put up there, as happened at most of the comparable health resorts of the time. Instead, Priessnitz housed in meagrely furnished peasants' cottages the patients who flocked to Gräfenberg from all parts of Austria and Prussia, and from the other countries around.

It would be difficult to list all the real and imaginary ailments that were treated by Priessnitz at Gräfenberg, for patients who went there could be suffering from apoplexy, asthma, cancer, concussion, epilepsy, gangrene, gout, impotence, melancholia, rheumatism, scrofula, syphilis, tropical decline, tuberculosis, or any other of the scores of diseases known in Europe at the time. Many of the patients would travel to Gräfenberg in style. E.S. Turner, in his illuminating book *Taking the Cure*, records that in 1839 Priessnitz's patients included twenty-two princes and princesses, one duke, one duchess, one hundred and forty-nine counts and countesses, eighty-eight barons and baronesses, fourteen generals, fifty-three staff officers, one hundred and ninety-six captains and subalterns, one hundred and four high and low civil servants, sixty-five divines, forty-six artists, and eighty-seven physicians and apothecaries.

On arriving at Gräfenberg, the patient would be shown a fountain set up by former visitors in gratitude for the relief they had had from Priessnitz's 'cures'. The fountain was dedicated to 'The Genius of Cold Water'. There was another tribute to Priessnitz's powers in the form of a monumental lion. The significance of this sculpture was explained by an inscription which suggested that man, having rejected water, a remedy that he shared with all animals, had been punished by becoming diseased and debilitated. By making the primitive virtues of water known again, the inscription went on, Priessnitz was infusing a new vigour into the human race.

Priessnitz made a point of attending the first bath taken by each patient. During this session, the Genius of Cold Water would look so closely at the patient's skin that there were many at Gräfenberg who said that Priessnitz 'could see inside you'. By the appearance of the patient's skin Priessnitz would know which of his many forms of treatment he ought to recommend.

In his early days at Gräfenberg, Priessnitz relied principally on comparatively simple 'wet sponge' treatments, but by 1840 he had developed several more drastic techniques. In the best-known of these, the patient would be wrapped tightly in a coarse linen sheet which would previously have been soaked in plenty of cold water. Over this, a thick quilt or blanket would be laid and, over that, an even thicker covering like an eiderdown or duvet. At first, the cold wet sheet that was nearest to the patient's skin would feel extremely uncomfortable, but this would soon be superseded by a delightful sensation of warmth and the patient would begin to perspire. The length of time that the patient would have to stay in the cocoon varied according to the nature and the seriousness of the case. Some patients were vigorously rubbed with wet sheets so that the resulting friction made their skin both red and warm. This, it was believed, had a specially stimulating effect on the person being so roughly massaged.

Among the more severe treatments that might be imposed at Gräfenberg on the patients were the 'sweating blanket', the use of which over a period of four or five hours induced a temporary fever; the 'plunge bath', which was a large tank of icy spring water in which a patient was breathtakingly immersed; the 'sitz bath', the bath that could be used for soaking the back of an aching head; and the 'ascending douche', which sent a jet of water vertically towards a patient's underside. Half a mile from the principal centre of treatment there were powerful cataracts under which male and female patients were subjected to the most exhilarating treatments of all. On a strong male patient for whom one of these 'cold douches' was prescribed, a column of water might be allowed to fall from a height of over eighteen feet. It is hardly surprising that one of these patients described the experience as being like receiving a beating from a great stick. The hardiest patients managed to stay under the jets for periods of up to one hour.

Priessnitz's aims – to drive out by the use of water all the bad and unwanted elements from the human system – were derided at first by most orthodox medical men, who regarded him as a crank or quack. But Priessnitz's rigorous system, combined with the limitations that he imposed on all detectable self-indulgence, undoubtedly produced some impressive results. John Gibbs, who spent four years at Gräfenberg, and whose letters from there were published in 1847, quoted police reports which showed that during the year 1843 there had been one thousand and fifty patients at the town, and that of these only four had died, two of the four having been declared by Priessnitz to be incurable. According to another source, seven thousand two hundred patients had come under Priessnitz's care between 1831 and 1841, and only thirty-eight of these had failed to survive his treatments.

The demonstrable success of Priessnitz's methods soon induced other people to set up similar water-based healing centres in other parts of Europe, but the majority of these enjoyed only a limited amount of popularity, and some were fated soon to disappear altogether. In Britain, however, Priessnitz's ideas were received with enthusiasm.

The two men principally responsible for introducing hydropathy to an English public – Doctor James Wilson and Doctor James Manby Gully – met during the 1830s when Doctor Gully was helping to edit some medical periodicals and Doctor Wilson was an occasional contributor. Both doctors disapproved of the exaggerated use of drugs fashionable then in some medical circles, and of the obsolescent practice of bleeding patients, which was not only useless, they felt, but was actually harmful. When Doctor Wilson, who had himself been suffering from a number of chronic complaints, returned to London from Gräfenberg ready to sing the praises of Priessnitz and his close-to-Nature therapeutic methods, he sought out his former colleague so that he could tell him of the advantages of the Silesian water cure.

At once, the two men decided to set up a resort, in England, that would be as effective as Gräfenberg, but which would be in surroundings that were a little less awesome, and which would have more civilised accommodation for its visitors than the austere and often smelly apartments provided for Priessnitz's patients. Such a place, they saw clearly, could be pleasantly profitable to its proprietors. When they had looked round a bit, they settled on the little Worcestershire town of Malvern as being the most suitable site for their activities.

Malvern – set on the side of an ancient range of hills that could be easily climbed and from which magnificent views could be obtained – had unusually pure waters, admirably clear air, and had been used as a spa of a minor kind for many years. It was not too far from London; it was not too near any of the recently developed factory towns. Within a very short time of making their mutual decision, Doctor Wilson had purchased the lease of the Crown Hotel at Malvern and had renamed it Gräfenberg House. Doctor Gully, co-operating at first rather than competing, had taken a large building called Tudor House. He was soon to acquire another, called Holyrood House, for the use of his female patients.

From the very start of their hydropathic activities on the slopes of the Malvern Hills, Doctors Wilson and Gully were regarded with the deepest distrust by the orthodox medical practitioners of the neighbourhood – 'The Water Quacks', they were called, by those who feared that their less loyal fee-paying patients would desert to the new arrivals. Both men managed to survive financially, however, and then both prospered exceedingly as hydropathy became, for a generation at least, 'all the rage'. Doctor Gully, who is said to have had a sympathetic and charming manner, did even better than his associate, for he was able to attract more rich and famous clients to Malvern than Doctor Wilson – possibly because Doctor Wilson, who regarded himself as a sensible dietitian, earned an unenviable reputation as a martinet. In time, as Doctor Wilson became increasingly jealous of the success of his former friend, relations between the two hydropaths became strained.

Malvern's drawing power increased after the railway reached the town in 1861, and then new hydropathic establishments, with younger and more energetic proprietors, appeared in all parts of the town. The English boom in wet-sheeting and cold-douching, which brought so much prosperity to Malvern, lasted until the more glamorous Continental watering places, patronized in such an extravagant fashion by the Prince of Wales, became altogether more attractive. Then the relatively modest hydropathic enterprises on the Worcestershire hillside started to fail, one by one, and the buildings that had seen so many cold water cures attempted were converted, in steadily increasing numbers, into hotels, boarding houses or schools. By the end of the nineteenth century only Priessnitz House, of all the Malvern hydropathic establishments, was still in operation, and even that had had to have its name changed to 'The County Hydropathy' because Priessnitz was dead and virtually forgotten, and Gräfenberg had lost its former appeal. Doctor Gully had lost much credit, too, through his connection with the notorious Charles Bravo scandal.

A small hydropathic establishment called Ben Rhydding was purpose-built on the Yorkshire moors at the height of the water-cure boom. It was sponsored, in the first instance, by an ex-Mayor of Leeds named Hamer Stansfield, who had been to Gräfenberg and, like Doctor Wilson, had returned to England convinced that Priessnitz's methods were little short of miracle-working. Every patient who went to Ben Rhydding paid high fees. Each was provided with a private bath, a rare luxury in those days, and there was a plunge bath and a douche on every floor. Further health-giving amenities at this palatial 'hydro' included a 'rain box' in which a patient could sit while a thousand piercing jets of water were fired at his or her body; vapour baths, in which the limbs of rheumaticky patients were made more flexible, hopefully, with steam; and a 'compressed air chamber' made from thick iron plates in which a patient could sit for up to two hours, while the pressure of the air that the tank contained was gradually increased until it was seven and a half pounds per square inch above normal. No alcoholic refreshments could be consumed by any of the patients at Ben Rhydding in the early days of the establishment. When the medical super-intendent, a Doctor William Maclecd, decided to relax this rule to pacify a number of his patients who had found the enforced deprivation intolerable, a number of the other patients, mostly members of the Society of Friends, are said to have walked out.

The development of the hydropathic spa at Matlock, in Derbyshire, is associated primarily with an extraordinary man, the energetic industrialist John Smedley, of Lea Mills. Born at Wicksworth in 1803, Smedley looked after the family spinning business through some very hard times until, by 1840, he had coaxed the mills into such a secure and prosperous state that he felt that he could take a holiday. So he went on a Grand Tour of Europe, but contracted a serious illness, due, it has been said, to his having spent too long in a cold damp church in Switzerland. For a time he was totally incapacitated. Then, when he had made a partial recovery, he started to wonder whether the troubles that had beset him might not be due to the 'awful folly of living for the gratifications of this life'. Sent by his doctors to take a cure at Ben Rhydding, Smedley, suffering acutely from the dis-comforts of his treatment there, then went through some form of religious exaltation in which he 'entered the fold of the Great Shepherd and experienced unbounding joy and confidence'. At once, he decided that he would return to Matlock and that he would devote the rest of his life to bringing all his employees willy-nilly to God and to showing them, if necessary by some form of compulsion, the advantages of hydropathy.

The workpeople at Lea Mills heard of their employer's proposals with some disquiet. They had suffered enough, they thought, when their boss had tried to make them all take

Fearn's Family Pills, but there were no trade associations at that time strong enough to protect them from their presiding zealot, and soon they were being urged to make use of the free water hospital that Smedley had opened in buildings adjacent to his mills. They were being cajoled or brow-beaten, too, into experimenting almost endlessly with packs, douches and other appliances for water treatment, whether they had anything actually wrong with them or not. A number of the unluckiest spinners were persuaded to walk barefoot, in winter, to a well that was at least half a mile away from the mills. As for the spiritual needs of the members of his little community, Smedley saw effectively to these by building a number of Methodist chapels and schoolrooms in the neighbourhood of the mills; by having at the mills a half-hour-long religious service each morning, which all his employees were required to attend; and by laying on at the mills large quantities of Bibles, which were stored in the general stock rooms along with the poultice materials, water bandages, and other items of equipment needed for the employees' physical regeneration.

Before long, news of John Smedley's animated campaign reached people in towns and villages that were quite a distance from Matlock, and many of the richer of these expressed their wish to share the hydropathic benefits that Smedley was conferring – with the greatest possible success, according to his own accounts – on the not wholly appreciative members of his staff. To accommodate the first wave of these eager visitors, Smedley and his wife, who appears to have approved wholeheartedly of what her husband was doing, were obliged to turn their house into a free hospital. They bought a house at Matlock Bath and took in patients, whom they asked to pay small fees. Later, they were obliged to enlarge this building, until it would accommodate a hundred patients at a time. These patients were willing to pay considerably higher fees for the privilege of staying at 'Smedley's Hydropathic' and for being shown how to take mustard baths, how to give themselves the 'wet silk gloves' treatment, and how to brace themselves for as many of the other idiosyncratic therapies devised by the Smedleys as they could bear. By 1862, Smedley had made a considerable fortune out of his varied activities – he had made so much money, in fact, that he was able to put up a huge castellated mansion, that he was to call 'Riber Castle', and it was here that he died. Smedley's Hydro ceased to be used as a hydropathic establishment soon after the First World War, but Matlock still attracts hundreds of visitors each year in its new rôle as a holiday resort and conference centre.

Derided as a pseudo-science by most members of the medical profession, resented by conventional pharmacists because its advocates did not believe in the use of drugs, and ridiculed by the recognized medical press (*The Lancet* sometimes indexed references to it under 'water death'), hydropathy in its purest form could hardly have been expected to survive. Even as public belief in Priessnitz's ideas dwindled, though, efforts were made to convince the less sophisticated that hydropathists really did have something of value to offer. Electrotherapy – the direction of electrical impulses to various parts of a patient's body so that muscular reactions could be stimulated – was introduced as an additional attraction at a number of hydropathic resorts. There were several variations on this basic technique. There was 'galvanism', in which an electric current would be passed through a patient's body after the current had been made to pass, first, through the body of an accredited attendant, and 'faradisation', in which a patient would be made to sit with his or her feet on a large electrode, while an attendant would apply another electrode to various parts of the patient's body. The last surviving hydropathists were given a small boost shortly after the end of the nineteenth century when the Curies, in France, announced to the world that they had managed to produce a tiny sample of radium. The managements of several of the surviving hydropathic establishments, and of at least two of the more respectable spas, were then quick to discover that the water used in their treatments was 'radioactive' and therefore almost magically beneficial to health.

Before the nineteenth century was much more than half over, Turkish baths were appearing as rapidly in various parts of Britain as hydropathic establishments had sprung up a decade or so before.[4] Modelled, loosely, on the original hot vapour baths opened in Brighton in 1784 by Sake Deen Mahomed, who had formerly been a surgeon with the East India Company, the later Turkish baths were opened to satisfy the demand prompted by the publication, in 1850, of David Urquhart's book *The Pillars of Hercules*. Descriptions in this book of the sensual delights to be experienced in the *hammams* of the East were accompanied by confident suggestions that exposure to the hot scented vapours of a *hammam* would heighten the bather's sensibilities and strengthen his or her bodily frame. 'The touch of your own skin is electric', reported Urquhart, writing on the after-effects of such a bath. 'The body thus renewed, the spirit wanders abroad and, reviewing its tenement, rejoices to find it clean and tranquil. There is an intoxication or dream that lifts you out of the flesh and yet a sense of life and consciousness that spreads through every member. Each breastful of air seems to pass not to the heart but to the brain and to quench not the pulsations of the one but the fancies of the other. That exaltation which requires the slumber of the senses – that vividness of sense that drowns the visions of the spirit – are simultaneously engaged in calm and unspeakable luxury; you condense the pleasures of many scenes and enjoy in an hour the existence of years'.

Turkish baths did – and do – undoubtedly produce the sensations suggested by Urquhart's purple prose. A few such baths were actually constructed, optimistically, inside lunatic asylums, but their popularity was to decline in Britain in time because they did not produce the therapeutic miracles that had been confidently predicted for them, and because too many of them were staffed by unskilled attendants who were liable to overbroil their clients, leaving them exhausted and apathetic. Orthodox medical men were not slow to warn their patients that the high temperatures to be found in Turkish baths might be dangerous to the heart. One of the few distinguished people to attempt to stem this ebb tide was the beautiful actress Lily Langtry, who wrote in 1885:

> I attribute my perfect health entirely to the Turkish Bath which I take twice a week regularly. I find it keeps my skin in excellent condition, notwithstanding the pigmentation one is unfortunately obliged to use on the stage, and I think for all small ailments the Turkish Bath is the best doctor to fly to.[5]

But Mrs Langtry was pleading in vain.

# The Birth of Tropical Medicine

*. . . Fear no more the heat o' the sun . . .*

WILLIAM SHAKESPEARE, *Cymbeline*

It was hard enough, in the nineteenth century, for those living in temperate climates to keep alive and in good health. Any journey that had to be made into the Tropics added fresh hazards to the dangers that had to be faced at home for malaria, yellow fever, and other unfamiliar diseases were rife. The story of the development of 'tropical medicine' is especially interesting because so many discoveries of prime importance in this field were made by so very few men.

One of the earliest of these was Patrick Manson, who, like so many more of the great medical innovators, was brought up in Scotland. His father – a local branch manager of the British Linen Bank – was moved to Aberdeen in 1857 when Patrick, his second son, was thirteen. Patrick was educated at the Gymnasium in that city and, later, at the West End Academy.

The plan was that the young man should become an engineer when he left school and he did, in fact, take up an apprenticeship with one of the local firms. Soon, however, he contracted some serious illness, and while he was convalescing from it he was encouraged to indulge his interest in natural history. Before long, he decided to give up the idea of making his living as an engineer. Instead, he said, he would like to take up the study of medicine at the University of Aberdeen.

By 1865, Manson had graduated with the degree of Bachelor of Medicine and he took his Doctorate in the following year. By that time, his elder brother was out in the Far East, and through his influence Manson was appointed by the Chinese Imperial Maritime Customs as their Medical Officer for Formosa. Manson stayed at Formosa for nearly five years. Then, when political unrest made it difficult for him to remain there any longer, he left the island and went to Amoy. There he took charge of a missionary society's hospital and dispensary and he built up an extensive private practice. There, too, he made his first really original and important observations.

The disease that is commonly known as 'elephantiasis' is a particularly unpleasant one, and a lot of people were suffering from it, at that time, in Amoy. In the early stages of the disease the flesh of the patient becomes inflamed, and this is followed by the development of granulamatous lesions, swellings and impaired circulation of the blood. The lymph glands then become enlarged and the lymph channels start to dilate. Over the years – if the condition is not treated – these channels then harden and become clogged with fibrous matter. Grotesque swellings follow, usually on the legs and scrotum, and the patient is compelled to carry around unsightly masses of tissue: as large, often, as footballs and occasionally larger even than that.

As Manson worked, surgically, to remove as many as possible of the massive tumours from which his patients were suffering, he was depressed by the apparent prevalence of the disease, and he was stimulated by the urgency of the need for finding some cure for it – or, better still, some method of prevention.

Manson's first chance to conduct his researches with any real success came after he had returned to Britain on leave in 1875. While he was in London, he was told that a man named Timothy Richards Lewis, working in Calcutta in 1870, had discovered, in the blood of patients who were suffering from elephantiasis, some minute thread-like worms or 'microfilariae'. When he returned to China, Manson made a series of observations which convinced him that there really was a close link between these filaria worms and the elephantoid diseases. Even more remarkable, he was able to show that the embryonic forms of the worm do not appear in the blood at all until sunset; that they then tend to increase in number until midnight; and that they then decrease in number until, by morning, they have virtually disappeared. What, he wondered, happened to the tiny filariae? How did they get out of the body?

Advancing a hypothesis that was little more than pure conjecture, Manson picked on the mosquito as the agent that most probably helped the embryos to escape. He based his guess on the erroneous assumption that the geographical areas in which mosquitos and filarial diseases are found are identical. Scientists have shown more recently that they are not. In a brave attempt to find out whether or not his assumption was correct, Manson started to feed mosquitos on a patient whose blood was teeming with embryonic *filariae*. 'After many months of work', he wrote in the 'China Customs Medical Reports' for September 1877, 'often following up false scents, I ultimately succeeded in tracing the filaria through the stomach wall into the abdominal cavity and then into the thoracic muscles of the mosquito. I ascertained that during this passage the little parasite increased enormously in size. It developed a mouth, an alimentary canal, and other organs . . . Manifestly, it was on the road to a new human host'.

Manson's discovery – that a parasite could pass part of its life in a human or animal host and part in the tissues of a blood-sucking insect – was of paramount importance in the history of the conquest of tropical disease. In the next stages of his research he was not quite so fortunate, for he made what he described as 'a regrettable mistake, the result of a want of books'. The mosquito, he reckoned, was short-lived. At the time of the insects' death, Manson's reasoning went on, the tiny filarial larvae inside it would probably pass by natural means into static water of some kind, and from there they would be taken up by their next human or animal host.

Manson's theory was ingenious, but the true story was even stranger than that.

The first hint that Manson needed came in 1883, when an anonymous reviewer, writing in the *Veterinarian* (*Volume LVI*) suggested that the parent worm might be introduced into its human or animal host by some agent, so far unidentified. Might not the worm be deposited in the host, the writer enquired, by the mosquito in the act of biting?

And that, as scientists in the world were soon to know, was what had been happening with unfortunate results for humanity for countless years. When a mosquito bit an infected human or animal, it would take into its own blood stream a number of microscopic but highly active embryos. These would pass their larval stage in the body of the biting insect, as Manson's initial investigations had shown. Introduced, then, by the mosquito in the act of biting into a new and larger host, the female worms would pass through their mature phase in that host, producing in the process large numbers of microscopic but highly active embryos. Some of these, in their turn, would be removed by a biting insect, and the cycle could be endlessly repeated.

Before the end of 1883, Manson had left Amoy and had settled in Hong Kong, where he quickly built up another private practice. He spent much of his time and energy here in public works, starting a school of medicine which was to become an important part of the University of Hong Kong. Three years later, he was awarded an honorary degree by the University of his home town, Aberdeen. This was the first time that his highly important scientific work had received any official recognition. Three years after that he retired from practice, returned to Britain from China, and decided to make his home in Scotland. His plans went wrong, though. Within a year Manson was driven, through certain financial losses, to take up medical practice again, this time in London. In 1892 he was appointed to the post of Physician to the Seamen's Hospital Society, and that gave him a chance to resume his researches into the causes of tropical diseases of various kinds.

During his time at the Seamen's Hospital, Manson began to ponder on the dreadful sufferings caused by malaria.

Malaria – otherwise called 'ague', 'intermittent fever', 'hill fever' and 'jungle fever' – was one of the first of the really dangerous infections to be positively identified by man. Records of it go back at least as far as the fifth century B.C. The disease, which had until modern times a world-wide incidence, was the cause of more sickness and death than any other. It is fairly easily recognised, because sufferers from it tend to be cut down, repeatedly and at fairly regular intervals, by severe paroxysms of chills and fever. These periodic attacks are usually accompanied by anaemia, enlargement of the spleen, and profuse sweating. Complications are liable to develop that often prove fatal. A fairly effective form of treatment of the disease had been discovered before the end of the seventeenth century, when the bark of the cinchona tree – known now in its prepared form as 'quinine' – had been found by the Jesuits at Lima to alleviate some of the worst of the disease's symptoms. The causes of the disease, though, were still unknown when Manson started work at the Seamen's Hospital.

For many years past, medical writers had been suggesting, without any positive evidence to prove their point, that mosquitos might have something to do with the spread of malaria. Then, in 1880, a parasite which looked as if it might cause malaria was isolated and identified by the French physician and pathologist Alphonse Laveran. Laveran, who had served as an army surgeon in the Franco-Prussian War of 1870–71, had been practising and teaching military medicine in Algiers when he made this most important discovery. In 1884, he had published the definitive work on the subject, calling it his *Treatise on the Marshy Fevers with a Description of the 'Microbes du paludisme'*. Marshes and swamps are notoriously the ideal places in which mosquitos can breed.

Manson considered Laveran's theories carefully. Then, the man who discovered that the development of the elephantiasis bloodworm occurred in the body of a mosquito proceeded to argue by analogy that the malaria parasite might develop, in more or less the same way, in the same irritating little host.

There were, Manson knew, certain forms of the malaria parasite which appeared when they were examined under the microscope to behave in an extraordinary way. They would develop movable filaments which could break off and move away independently through the surrounding blood fluid. Manson was much too experienced to believe that Nature had provided these filaments unnecessarily. Surely, he argued, they were meant to fulfil some useful purpose. Could such a filament, he wondered, be intended to break off and start a life of its own while the parasite of which it had been part was in the body of some intermediate host, such as the stomach of a mosquito?

While Manson was still pondering on these lines, a young man named Ross, on leave in England from India, was introduced to him. Ronald Ross had been born at Almora, a hill station in the North-West Provinces of India, on 13 May 1857. His father, General Campbell Claye Grant Ross of the Indian Army, had sired nine more children after Ronald. The family was financially comfortable, and every member of it seems to have been more than usually talented or to have had some exceptional intellectual endowment. When he was eight, Ronald Ross had been sent to Britain to be educated. He went, first, to two small schools at Ryde in the Isle of Wight. Then in 1869 he had been moved to a boarding school at Springhill, near Southampton, where he had been encouraged to spend his spare time in such pursuits as zoology and studying the elementary laws of harmony. When he was old enough to leave school he had thought that he would like to become an artist, but his father had other ideas. In deference to his father's views, Ross had become a medical student at St Bartholomew's Hospital. Unfortunately he had found the work at 'Bart's' disagreeably difficult, and by the end of his time there, he had failed to obtain sufficient qualifications to enable him to practise as a doctor. He had managed, however, in 1879, to pass the M.R.C.S. examination, which qualified him to take the relatively humble job of ship's surgeon. He had gone away in that capacity for four or five leisurely voyages, during which he had spent much of his time writing plays in blank verse, and a novel.

By 1881, Ross had managed to pass some more examinations and had been able, then, to enter the Indian Medical Service. For several years after that, he had held temporary appointments with various regiments serving in Madras, and at a succession of station hospitals. He had found the sunlight and clear air of India extraordinarily invigorating, he recalled later, and having a lot of free time in which he could follow non-medical pursuits of various kinds he had studied the French, German, and Italian languages; he had read widely in the world's poets and in the classics; and he had become seriously interested in mathematics. He had taken a Diploma in Public Health and he had studied some elementary bacteriology, but there was little to suggest, at that time, that he might be any more interested in medicine than he was in any of the other subjects in which he was dabbling.

Once he had met Patrick Manson, though, Ross was a changed man. He was almost literally 'inspired' by Manson. In the following year, 1895, he returned to India determined to solve the problem of the causes of malaria. Through him, Manson seemed to be working vicariously.

A little more than two years later, on 20 August 1897, Ross made his first significant advance: he found, in the gastrointestinal tract of a mosquito of one particular kind, the pigmented oocysts, or filaments, of the malaria parasite.

To appreciate fully the long odds against this discovery, one has to remember that there are about 250 different species of the mosquito family. Most of the females in these species need a meal of blood before they can bring their eggs to maturity. To obtain this blood, they have elongated probosces which they can drive down through the skins of the victims of their choice. Having found blood and having sucked it in, they lay their eggs on some convenient water surface, the water being, for preference, stagnant. The eggs hatch out to produce small aquatic larvae or 'wrigglers' which move themselves about under the water surface by making sharp jerks with their bodies, and which manage to keep themselves alive by eating algae and other minute organisms. In one of the species that breed like this Ronald Ross managed to find what he was looking for: the all-important filaments, in a mosquito called, now, by scientists Anopheles.

Anopheles mosquitos, which are very special, can be readily recognised by the position in which they habitually come to rest: an Anopheles mosquito, inactive, will normally keep its proboscis, head and body in a straight line, and at an angle to the surface on which it is resting. Its wings are spotted in a distinctive way. The fact that Ross was not a trained observer – was, indeed, very far from being one – makes it all the more extraordinary that he should have made one of the most significant discoveries in the history of medical research.

By the following year, after he had made a thorough study of Protesoma, a parasite found in the blood of birds suffering from a disease comparable to human malaria, Ross had with certainty established the fact that malaria is an infectious disease transmitted from man to man by the mosquito. He had shown, therefore, that it is not, as it had been up to that time almost universally believed, contracted from the air or from water. Meanwhile an American researcher, W.G. MacCullum of Baltimore, had established what the moving filaments associated with the malaria parasite really were: they were male elements, and they were intended to fertilise the female forms of the parasite which had no such motile elements. On 28 July 1898 Manson told the members of the British Medical Association, meeting at Edinburgh, of Ross's important discovery. The news was received with intense interest. Honours of various kinds were showered on Ross from many different parts of the world. One of the earliest of these was the offer of a post as a lecturer at the School of Tropical Medicine in Liverpool. Ross accepted the offer, and returned to England from India in February 1899. Three years later, he was given a Professorship. In 1902 he was awarded the Nobel Prize for Medicine and was appointed a Companion of the Bath.

During the years that followed his establishment in England, Ross worked continuously and with the greatest energy towards the complete eradication of malaria throughout the world. He intended to do this through the total destruction of the Anopheles mosquito from all parts of the world, by eliminating all the sites in which it might possibly breed; by the application of films of oil to the surfaces of all sheets of water which might possibly be breeding places and which could not be eliminated, so that the breathing tubes of all mosquito 'wrigglers' that might be found in those waters would be fatally clogged; and by the use of the few larvicides available at the time. The task Ross had set himself was a huge one, and it could not possibly be accomplished in one man's lifetime. But by the time the Ross Institute and Hospital for Tropical Diseases had been founded in his honour, in 1926, on Putney Heath, and he had been made the Director-in-Chief of it, his recommendations had been taken seriously in nearly every part of the world. In no other way could mankind rid itself of the most troublesome of all the diseases of the tropics.

Unfortunately for Ross, he was not able to concentrate on his aims with complete single-mindedness, for before he had been busy for many months on his historic campaign he became involved in a bitter controversy with the Italian scientist Battista Grassi and his colleagues.

Grassi, it appeared, had been trying to solve the problems of malaria at approximately the same time as Ross, and the argument was about which of the men had actually been the first to arrive at the correct answer. The weakness in Ross's case lay in the fact that it was Grassi and not himself who had successfully established the complete sequence of steps in the life cycle of the parasite that causes human malaria. The extraordinary way in which the embryonic parasite passes from the gastro-enteric tract of the mosquito, through its thoracic wall, and into its proboscis, ready for injection into an innocent 'victim', had not been precisely ascertained by Ross, though only a fully trained and most meticulous scientist would have noticed any gap in his observations. Undeterred by the acrimonious comments made by his Italian 'rivals', Ross continued his Herculean labours with the full approval of his mentor, Patrick Manson.

During the last twenty-five years of his life, Manson was loaded heavily with honours and responsibilities. In 1897, he was asked to act as the Chief Physician and Medical Adviser to the Colonial Office, and in this capacity he was able to bring some strong influence to bear on Joseph Chamberlain, who was at that time Secretary of State for the Colonies. Appalled by the comparative ignorance of tropical medicine of nearly all the medical practitioners who had gone out to serve in Britain's equatorial territories, Manson drew up a scheme for the systematic instruction of students in the diagnosis, treatment and prevention of tropical disease. In 1898 he published his *Tropical Diseases: a Manual of the Diseases of Warm Climates* – a masterly work based on his huge experience, and containing many references to the original researches he had made while he had been in China. The foundation of the London School of Tropical Medicine, in 1899, was the direct outcome of his efforts. At the International Congress of Medicine held in London in 1913, Manson, by that time Sir Patrick, was described as The Father of Tropical Medicine, an honour that he indisputably deserved.[1]

Yellow Fever, or 'Yellow Jack' – a dreaded sickness which had its chief seats in Central America and in the coastal territories of West Africa – remained during the whole of the nineteenth century one of the chief scourges of the Tropics. Frequently, this horrible disease would be referred to as 'Vomito Negro', since the sufferer's vomit would all too often be black with blood, which would usually herald the death of the patient. Work on the construction of the Panama

Canal, started by De Lesseps in 1882, had to be abandoned soon after it was begun owing to the prevalence of yellow fever in the territories through which the Canal was to pass.

In the year 1900 there were 1400 cases of yellow fever in Havana alone. By that time, though, the possibility that the mosquito might be the carrier of the disease had been suggested, and the American Army Board had been instructed to investigate the matter. Led by a courageous doctor called Walter Reed, members of the Board went to Havana on a mission that was to prove historic.

The chief difficulty that faced the members of the mission arose from the fact that it had not been possible up to that time to transmit the disease to any animal. If any experiments were to be carried out, human volunteers would have to be found who would be willing to face the hazards associated with this horrible sickness. The first member of the Board to submit to being bitten by what was believed to be an infected mosquito, James Carroll, did in fact suffer an attack of the fever but was fortunate enough to survive. It was Carroll, later, who found that the disease could be transmitted by the injection of blood or serum from an infected person, without a mosquito having necessarily to be involved as the agent.

Other vitally important facts were established, too, by members of the mission. Seven men who volunteered to sleep in the bedclothes of patients who had been suffering from yellow fever failed to develop the disease because they were not bitten by any mosquito. This seemed to show that the disease could not be communicated from one human being to another except by some form of inoculation. When it was shown that the disease could be transmitted by the injection of blood or serum that had been carefully filtered, proof seemed to have been obtained that the fever was, in fact, caused by a virus of some kind.

As soon as the mosquito's part in spreading yellow fever had been indisputably demonstrated, William C. Gorgas, the Chief Sanitary Officer of Havana, instituted a dynamic campaign against the little winged vectors. This, he hoped, would clear his territories of the pestilence. He began by isolating carefully every single yellow fever patient under his jurisdiction, and by screening each of the fever sufferers so thoroughly that no mosquito could possibly get access to him or her. By this means, Gorgas argued, the insects flying about Havana would be prevented from becoming infected with the fever. He was right. Within three months, Havana had been virtually cleared of the fever for the first time since medical records had been kept. Work on the Panama Canal could be restarted, and it was completed by 1914.

The campaign against yellow fever, conducted so brilliantly and with such memorable dedication, was not to be allowed to continue without some notable human casualties. In the early days at Havana, for instance, J. W. Lazear, one of the members of the Army Board, died from yellow fever contracted from having been accidentally bitten by an infected mosquito. The leading Japanese bacteriologist Hideyo Noguchi succumbed similarly in 1928 in Africa, where he was travelling in an endeavour to identify the causative organism of the disease. A third victim, Adrian Stokes, managed to show before he, too, perished with the fever that certain Asiatic Rhesus monkeys could be successfully inoculated with the organisms that caused the malady. This was a great step forward, because it meant that human volunteers would no longer be needed for imperative research.

African sleeping sickness is a disease that should not be confused with the disorder *Encephalitis Lethargica*, or 'sleepy sickness', which is found principally in Europe and other places that have temperate climates. During the nineteenth century, the African disorder was one of the most serious of all the ailments suffered by inhabitants of that Continent. It dealt with its victims slowly, making them undergo, as they wasted away, long bouts of fever, during which they became increasingly lethargic, until they had literally no life at all.

One of the first men to do anything really remarkable about the African sleeping sickness was David Bruce, from

New Zealand. Bruce had been investigating a strange disease called 'nagama' that affected cattle, causing them to become feverish and anaemic, so that they wasted away and eventually died. In the blood of some of the beasts suffering from this disease, Bruce had found minute organisms of the kind known as trypanosomes. By 1894, he was able to show that the trypanosomes were being carried to the domestic cattle by the tsetse fly, *Glossina Morsitans*. The tsetse fly got the trypanosomes in the first instance, said Bruce, from wild animals of the big game variety. This, he contended, was proved by the fact that where there was no big game, there was no nagama.

Investigations were carried on after that by three members of a Royal Society Commission who went out to Africa to find out what they could about the serious outbreaks of sleeping sickness that were happening in Uganda. One of the three, Aldo Castellani, was a graduate of the University of Florence and had been trained, later, at the London School of Tropical Medicine. In 1902, Castellani happened to find in the cerebrospinal fluid of patients suffering from sleeping sickness trypanosomes of the kind to which David Bruce had drawn the attention of the veterinary world. Could tsetse flies, wondered Castellani, be acting as the carriers of the organisms that caused this debilitating and normally fatal disease?

By establishing the geographical distribution of as many sufferers from sleeping sickness as possible, and by relating his findings to the approximate geographical distribution of the various species of tsetse fly, Castellani was able to conclude that the insect known by scientists as *Glossina Palpalis* was the vector of the unwanted and usually fatal parasites.

After that, drastic action had to be taken, as thorough as the campaign that had virtually eradicated the yellow fever from Havana. Unfortunately for those who had to take the action, they found it extermely difficult under the circumstances prevailing at the time to destroy the flies which were mostly in impenetrable jungle thickets. Nor was it very much easier to move all sleeping sickness sufferers from the 'fly areas' so that the infected flies could die out harmlessly, to be replaced, in the ordinary course of Nature, by flies that were free from the unwanted trypanosomes. Always, it seemed, there would be a number of self-centred and unreasonable sufferers who would refuse to be moved away from the homes in which they wished to die, or even worse, would hide themselves away in secret and inaccessible places where only hungry tsetse flies could get at them. Enthusiasts who suggested that the entire wild animal population of the affected territories should be wiped out met with a cool response from big game hunters, naturalists, conservationists and others. Only, it seemed, when the whole of the tropical areas of Africa had been properly reclaimed and were being intensively cultivated would the dangerous tsetse fly be rendered harmless. And what hope was there of that?

In areas that were less vast and more readily manageable, campaigns for the destruction of the unwanted tsetse fly stood a greater chance of success. One such operation was mounted during the years 1911–13 in the Portugese island of Principe, off the West Coast of Africa. First, the thickets and undergrowth were cleared, and all those suffering from the disease were screened carefully so that they were quite inaccessible to the flies. Then, a team of ten men was asked to walk, in pairs, through the infested clearings. Each man wore white clothes and protective headgear and carried on his back a square piece of dark cloth that had been thickly smeared with the sticky substance known as bird lime. Four hundred and seventy thousand tsetse flies, tempted to settle on these ingeniously contrived traps, were caught and destroyed. Before long, Principe had been completely cleared of a pestilence which had been the cause of one-third of the total deaths on the island.

# 13

# *The Treatment of the Mentally Sick in the Nineteenth Century*

*. . . Babylon in all its desolation is a sight not so*
*awful as that of the human mind in ruins . . .*

SCROPE BERDMORE DAVIES (d. 1852)
*From a Letter to Thomas Raikes*

Medical and institutional treatment given to insane persons before the last years of the eighteenth century was callous, to say the least: at the Bethlehem Hospital in London, for example, the lunatics were kept in unheated cells and were exhibited to members of the general public much as animals are still exhibited in zoos. Frequently, the patients would have to suffer positive brutality, being kept in severe forms of restraint such as fetters and strait-jackets, and all too often being whipped, immersed in icy water, or maltreated in some other way. By a strange coincidence, two of the first men to suggest that the insane should be treated as suffering humans rather than as savage beasts were working along more or less the same lines at the same time in two different countries, England and France, without either being aware of what the other was doing.

The Englishman, William Tuke, was born in York on 24 March 1732. Members of the Tuke family had been living in York for at least three generations, and they had included some of the earliest converts to Quakerism, William's parents being prominent members of the Society of Friends. Although William was to spend most of his life looking after the family business – the Tukes were wholesale tea and coffee merchants of considerable prosperity – he spent much of his time outside business hours in philanthropic works.

During 1791, it happened that another York member of the Society of Friends died in the County Asylum in circumstances that gave rise to suspicions that the death was due to maltreatment. William Tuke came to the conclusion that an institution 'for the care and proper treatment of those labouring under that most afflictive dispensation – the loss of reason' was urgently needed. In the spring of 1792 he brought to the notice of the members of the Society of Friends in Yorkshire his belief that the treatment of the insane ought to be radically altered. With the support of his son Henry, who had been working with him in the family business and who had been made in his twenty-fifth year a Minister of the Society of Friends, he proposed that a building should be put up that would accommodate thirty insane persons. The inmates, he said, should be treated on new, humane lines. They should not be subjected to any unnecessary restraints, and they should not be made to suffer whippings or any other irksome forms of discipline. Instead, the place should have, as far as possible, a quiet and orderly atmosphere and some forms of light industrial employment should be provided for the patients who were capable of profiting from them.

The Tukes and their associates had some difficulty at first in raising the necessary funds but eventually, in 1796, the York 'Retreat' was opened for the reception of patients. The inscription on the foundation stone of the home – *Hoc fecit amicorum caritas in humanitatis argumentum*[1] – set the tone for all the work of the establishment, and William Tuke was to live to see his revolutionary ideas abundantly justified, the success of his experiment being recognized not only in Yorkshire but in many other parts of the world. Ferrus, physician to Napoleon I, was to write of The Retreat that it was the first English asylum which deserved the attention of foreigners.

In France, meanwhile, a physician named Philippe Pinel had been advocating a new approach to the controversial subject of mental diseases. Pinel had been born at Saint-André, Tarn, in 1745, and he had arrived in Paris just eleven

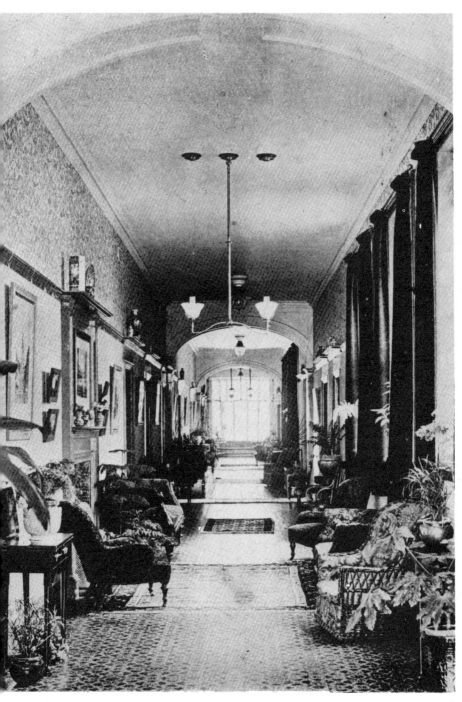

The interior of York Retreat

years before the Revolution. Having been friendly with Benjamin Franklin, the American scientist and publicist, and having learned from him the value of a scientific and logical approach to all human problems, Pinel had considered, for a time, emigrating instead to America. By 1787 he had started to write constructively about mental diseases. Then, in 1792, he was appointed to head the staff of the Bicêtre.

Part of the Hospice Générale set up on the left bank of the Seine by Cardinal Mazarin in 1656 and placed under the relatively humane supervision of Vincent de Paul, the Bicêtre was intended, in the first place, for destitute and infirm men. The women and prostitutes who needed to be rescued were accommodated in another part of the hospital known as 'La Salpêtrière', which had got its name from the original group of buildings put up there as a powder magazine during the reign of Louis XIII: the 'Petit Arsenal-Salpêtrière'. By the eighteenth century, the Salpêtrière had become the largest asylum in Europe, accommodating as many as eight thousand patients at a time. It contained infirmaries for the aged, the chronically ill, the paralysed, and – most distressing to visit of all – for the mentally defective. The demented women had been kept, for many decades, in fetters in insanitary cells where they were frequently attacked by rats.

As soon as Philippe Pinel was appointed to the Bicêtre, he let it be known that he intended to improve the conditions of the patients there. 'Are you crazy yourself, Citizen, that you want to unchain these animals?'[2] asked an official who went with him to look at his new charges. When Pinel replied that he was convinced that the mentally sick were distressed, primarily, because they were deprived of fresh air and liberty, the official is said to have shrugged his shoulders and to have exclaimed 'Do as you please!'[3] Shortly after that Pinel, who took – or appeared to take – no real interest in politics, was rescued from an angry revolutionary crowd by a former soldier whom he had released after ten years in chains. In 1794 he was appointed to administer the whole Salpêtrière, and here too he introduced his new and relatively humane approach to his charges. A painting hanging in the lecture theatre of the hospital shows him supervising the removal of the chains from the patients in 'Les Loges des Folles', an act which effectively reversed the methods favoured by doctors for centuries. For the rest of his long life, Pinel strove to make the Salpêtrière a place where as many distinguished men as possible could carry out all the research and curative work of which they were capable. His own *Nosographie Philosophique* published in 1798 contains descriptions of mental illnesses that are as simple and as accurate as anything written on the subject up to that time.

Back in Yorkshire, during the early years of the nineteenth century, various members of the Tuke family were able to continue and even augment the good work started by William and his son Henry. Samuel Tuke, Henry's son, was one of the most dedicated of these. Born in 1784, Samuel Tuke was persuaded by his father, as soon as he was old enough, to enter the family business, but this did not prevent him from making, in his spare time, an intensive study of medical literature. Before he was twenty-one, Samuel Tuke was corresponding with Thomas Hancock, who was later to become Physician to the City and Finsbury Dispensaries, on the subject of the influence of joy in mental diseases and related conditions. By 1809, he had resolved to collect all the information that was then available on the theory of insanity, on the treatment of the insane, and on the construction of asylums. Whenever he could, he would find out by personal inspection the conditions under which insane people were kept in various localities, noting, particularly, the abuses. In 1811, Tuke contributed two short papers to *The Philanthropist*, 'On the state of the Insane Poor' and 'On the Treatment of those Labouring Under Insanity, drawn from the Experience of The Retreat', and these articles are believed to have given the earliest known account of the consistent application of humane ideas to the treatment of insanity.

Impressed by his son's scholarly achievements, Henry Tuke suggested that Samuel should produce and publish a definitive account of the work that was being done at The Retreat. After two years of careful preparation, Samuel's *Description* was published in 1813. The book, and the work done at the Friends' asylum, were both praised highly by Sydney Smith in the Edinburgh Review, but other people were rather more critical. Among these were many officials connected with the unreformed madhouses of the period, one of whom – the physician of the York County Asylum – actually wrote an anonymous letter to a local newspaper defending the old system of 'caring for' lunatics, and this raised a violent controversy. The debate continued until Godfrey Higgins, a Yorkshire philanthropist who was keenly interested in the problems of the insane, and who was determined to get better treatment for them, managed, with the active support of the members of the Tuke family, to get some much-needed reforms carried out at the County Asylum.

William Tuke, the aged head of the family, had by that time lost his sight, but he was still managing to do much lively and useful work. In 1822, when he was ninety, he suffered a fatal paralytic seizure. Five years after that, Samuel Tuke, who had married a Miss Priscilla Hack of Chichester, became the father of twin boys, one of whom died within a few hours of his birth. The other boy – to be named 'Daniel Hack Tuke' – was delicate, and this impeded his education. Eventually, the young Daniel was apprenticed to a Bradford solicitor, but he found the work uncongenial and his health suffered. So in 1847, yet one more Tuke entered the service of The Retreat at York. Daniel spent two years there, studying in his spare time as much of the existing literature on insanity as he could. In 1850, he entered as a student at St Bartholomew's Hospital, London, and won several prizes. Two years later, he became a member of the Royal College of Surgeons and in 1853 he was awarded the degree of Doctor of Medicine by the University of Heidelberg. Next year, he was awarded a prize offered by the Association for Improving the Condition of the Insane.

Daniel Hack Tuke was internationally regarded, after that, as one of the world's greatest experts on the treatment of the insane. He travelled widely to visit asylums abroad and to record his observations of them, and was appointed, successively, Visiting Physician to the York Retreat, Examiner in Mental Philosophy to the University of London, Lecturer on Mental Diseases at the Charing Cross Hospital, and Governor of London's Royal Bethlehem Hospital. One of the most notable publications that resulted from Daniel Hack Tuke's prolonged investigations into the treatment of the insane in foreign countries and the colonies was a book about the asylums of the United States and Canada which appeared in 1885. The author was so scathing about some of the things he had seen in the Province of Quebec that investigations were set on foot and vast improvements followed.

Although Philippe Pinel worked almost ceaselessly, during his long years of superintendence, to improve the conditions under which his patients were housed at the Salpêtrière, treating every patient as an individual, with an individual's personal problems, it would be wrong to pretend that his idealistic aims were wholly achieved during his lifetime. As late as 1838, the most violent maniacs in the Salpêtrière were still required to sleep on the ground, and the helpless, lying on straw and all too carelessly nursed, were still liable to be attacked by hungry rats. Conditions in the place had not been much improved, though the rats seem at last to have been banished, when in 1856 a young man named Jean-Martin Charcot qualified as a *Médecin des Hôpitaux de Paris* and was almost immediately after offered a post as a junior consulting physician at the Salpêtrière.

During his first six years at the Salpêtrière, Charcot did some thorough research into a wide variety of medical subjects such as typhoid fever, rheumatism, and chronic pneumonia, but he showed no real inclination to specialise in disorders of the mind. Medical text books of the time devoted a few pages only to such topics as degenerative, infectious and vascular diseases of the brain, and to brain tumours, which were inaccurately classified. Chorea, epilepsy, and tetanus were given quite inadequate descriptions. In 1862 Charcot was appointed to the post that Pinel had held earlier in the century, and he became the Salpêtrière's Chief Physician. He was compelled to make an especially careful survey of the five thousand distressed persons who had been brought under his personal care and protection. Nearly half of his patients were insane. If they were not actually mad, they were epileptic, mentally disturbed, or just unable to cope with the problems of everyday life. Charcot, undiscouraged, embarked on an immensely difficult task. He tried to examine, methodically, each and every one of his charges. He tried to find out what was wrong with each, and he tried to tell his assistants how every individual patient should be cared for and if possible how each could be cured. But he did not try like his predecessors to cope with his numerous patients in the hospital's noisy and overcrowded wards. Instead, he would have them brought to his office, a small room illuminated by a single window. There were no furnishings of any consequence in the room: only a table, a few chairs, and a cupboard. All the wall and ceiling surfaces of the room, and the furniture it contained, were painted, dramatically, black. Charcot's personal appearance would not have been out of place on the stage. He 'was almost uncanny in the way he went straight to the root of the evil, often apparently after a rapid glance at the patient from his cold eagle eyes', reported Axel Munthe, author of the best-selling *Story of San Michele*, who in his youth had studied at the Salpêtrière. A detailed account of a typical consultation conducted by Charcot can be found in Georges Guillain's biography of the great clinician. The patient, says Guillain, would be taken to Charcot who would be sitting in his office. Then, Charcot would listen carefully while a clinical description of the case would be given to him by an intern:

> Then there was a long silence, during which Charcot looked, kept looking at the patient while tapping his hand

on the table. His assistants, standing close together, waited anxiously for a word of enlightenment. Charcot continued to remain silent. After a while he would request the patient to make a movement; he would induce him to speak; he would ask that his reflexes be examined and that sensory responses be tested. And then again silence, the mysterious silence of Charcot. Finally he would call for a second patient, examine him like the first one, call for a third patient, and always without a word, silently make comparisons between them.

This type of meticulous clinical scrutiny, particularly of a visual type, was at the root of all Charcot's discoveries. The artist in him, who went hand in hand with the physician, played an interesting part in these discoveries.[4]

Best known, perhaps, of all Charcot's earlier discoveries were those that he made in the field of pathological anatomy. Few hospitals, in those days, had laboratory facilities of the type that are regarded as essential today, but Charcot saw that at the Salpêtrière he would need at least one room that could be dedicated to research. He began by equipping, with a few microscopes, a room at the end of the cancer ward. Then he practically filled it with glass containers in which anatomical specimens could be preserved. Soon after that, he engaged a freelance research worker, Duchenne de Boulogne, who was an expert in the new and exciting field of medical photography. As Duchenne was interested, too, in electrophysiology, and was eager to find out as much as he could about the electrical excitation of human muscles, Charcot found that he had taken on to his staff an unexpectedly useful and forward-looking assistant.

Invaluable, too, was Charcot's friend and contemporary Edmé-Félix Alfred Vulpian, who was invited by Charcot to help with the immense task of examining and classifying all the patients in the Salpêtrière. As they worked, Charcot and Vulpian became increasingly aware of the tremors from which many of their patients were suffering. In some instances, the two men saw, these tremors could be shown to result directly from the distressing condition known variously as 'shaking palsy', 'paralysis agitans' and, more recently, 'Parkinson's disease'. In only a few cases, they found, were the tremors solely the result of old age. Could there be some disease other than the 'shaking palsy' that produced chronic tremors, Charcot and Vulpian wondered? After nearly two years of the most careful research, they decided that there was such a disease, and they gave it the name 'multiple sclerosis'. Earlier medical researchers had noticed that some deceased sufferers, when dissected, appeared to have in their nervous systems abnormal structures, labelled for convenience 'pathological plaques'. No one before Charcot and Vulpian had ever suggested that these 'plaques' might have some direct connection with a relatively common nervous disorder. By associating the 'plaques' directly with their 'new' disease multiple sclerosis, and by showing that the 'shaking palsy' was a quite different disease with an entirely different cause, Charcot and Vulpian made their names known in the more advanced medical circles in all parts of the civilised world.

By 1865, Charcot had added considerably to his international fame by some notable observations he had made when he was examining patients affected by the distressing neurosyphilitic condition known as 'tabes dorsalis' or 'locomotor ataxia'. With this the patient suffers intense pain, lack of muscular coordination, and wasting. Many of these patients, Charcot found, had distinctive lesions of the bones and joints. Accordingly he drew the attention of the medical world to these anatomical changes, choosing a medical congress in London as the right place to announce his important discoveries. The British doctors, properly impressed, gave the name 'Charcot's Joint' to the phenomenon noticed by their guest from over the Channel. Charcot's masterly description of the changes he had noticed in his 'tabes dorsalis' patients has never been bettered. His exceptional skills as a teacher and the international reputation he had earned by his researches brought students to the Salpêtrière from many different parts of the world, and these eager pupils were privileged to witness the great Frenchman's investigations into the nature of hysteria and the neuroses.

Until Charcot started these researches, no one had attempted very seriously to examine the disorders of the nervous system for which no positive organic basis could be suggested: the 'mental illnesses', that is, that did not appear to be due to some physical defect of the brain or of the nerves, or to some identifiable chemical or toxic cause. Way back in the seventeenth century, Thomas Sydenham (1624–89) had referred to hysteria as 'the Proteus that cannot be laid hold of'. Charcot's views were just as graphically expressed:

> Epilepsy, chorea, hysteria . . . come to us like so many Sphinxes . . . symptomatic combinations deprived of anatomical substratum do not present themselves to the mind of the physician with that appearance of solidity, of objectivity, of affections connected with an appreciable organic lesion.
>
> There are even some who see in some of these affections only an assemblage of odd incoherent phenomena inaccessible to analysis, and which had better, perhaps, be banished to the category of the unknown. It is hysteria which especially comes under this sort of proscription.[5]

Charcot's researches into the disorders that had mystified so many medical men were given a real urgency around the year 1870. By that time, one of the ancient buildings of the Salpêtrière had become so dilapidated that it seemed likely to fall down. In this building there were accommodated patients of many different kinds – the clearly and permanently insane being lodged there without any attempt having been made to separate them from the epileptics and the hysterics, whose troubles were, in the main, episodic. Once the hospital authorities had realised that the building would have to be evacuated, Charcot decided that as he was the Senior Physician he ought to take into his own immediate care all those displaced patients who were not indisputably and incurably insane.

The task of separating the patients into recognizably different classes was one for which Charcot, with his previous clinical experience, was peculiarly well fitted. From the start, he divided the patients coming into his new 'Epileptic Quarters' into three principal categories: the true sufferers from epilepsy, who were liable to have such serious seizures, and so often, that they could not safely be let out of hospital; the sufferers from neuroses and hysterias of various kinds; and the epileptics who were also neurotic or hysterical.

From ancient times and until quite recently, hysteria – a state of over-anxiety characterized by excessive laughter or crying – had been thought by most doctors to be an exclusively feminine disorder, caused, as far as anyone could tell, by some abnormal movement of the uterus. Aretaeus, who practised in the first century A.D., had stated with certainty that the uterus was liable to rise suddenly in the abdominal cavity, bringing unaccustomed pressure to bear on the vital organs which caused agitation, breathlessness, choking, and, finally, unconsciousness. Medical practitioners throughout the Middle Ages had tended to treat hysteria with techniques such as invocation and exorcism which were intended to persuade the wandering womb to return to its proper place in the patient's body. During the decades that immediately preceded Charcot's researches into hysteria, however, some more enlightened workers had been attempting to dispel the clouds of ignorance and superstition with which the subject had for so long been surrounded. In 1837, for instance, Sir Benjamin Collins Brodie, who had been trained partly at the Hunterian School in Great Windmill Street, London, and who had assisted at an operation on King George IV for the removal of a tumour from the royal scalp, published his lectures on some local nervous affections. In these lectures, the royal Sergeant-Surgeon had examined such phenomena as the occurrence of hysterical pains in women, and the frequency with which a hysterical patient's knees would become stiff. This manifestation was to be known, after that, as 'Brodie's knee'. Eighteen years after that, some further observations on the subject had been published by Charcot's own assistant Duchenne de Boulogne and these had been followed, in 1859, by a scholarly book called *The Clinical and Therapeutic Treatment of Hysteria* that had been written by one of Charcot's senior colleagues, Pierre Briquet. Charcot thought highly of Briquet's work, paying him, in a lecture, this frank tribute: 'Briquet . . . established beyond dispute that hysteria is governed in the same way as other morbid conditions by rules and laws, which attentive and sufficiently numerous observations always permit us to establish'.[6] But it was Charcot himself who set out to make members of the medical profession generally aware of the different forms that hysteria might take, stressing, in the process, the more unusual signs and symptoms of this disturbance that can be all too easily missed. Characteristically, he insisted on subdividing these forms into convulsive attacks and non-convulsive attacks. In the first of these, he showed, the patient would receive certain well-authenticated warning signs such as palpitations, feelings of tightness in the head, and the unmistakable choking sensation known as 'globus hystericus' which gave the patient the same kind of discomfort as would a ball pressing upwards in the throat. After that, the patient would pass into a second phase, in which he or she would probably fall backwards and would become unconscious, would swell at the neck, and would usually foam at the mouth. A few minutes later, the 'tonic' phase would follow, in which the patient's arms and legs would be motivated by short but most disturbing twitchings. Muscular relaxation would be restored, after that, together with more or less normal breathing. The patient might then perform grotesque movements, and in many cases would go on to act out some at least of his or her feelings:

Pleasure, pain, fear, even fright, love, hatred etc.; not infrequently this sentiment and mimicry are in relation to a vivid impression or an emotion formerly experienced by the patient, which often has played a part in the explosion of hysterical symptoms. In such cases we sometimes see the patient recall a whole scene in his former life (some dispute, accident, etc.). Mimicry mostly takes the first place, but some patients also scream in connection with their sentiments, and some make long speeches.[7]

Usually, the attack would end at that point, and the patient would slowly recover. Charcot's observations were used for several decades after that in the instruction of students. As he carried out his researches into 'La Grande Hystérie', as Charcot and his associates decided to call the severest form of attack in which most of the features he had observed were manifested, the great man noticed that many of the patients in his epilepsy-hysteria wards had frequent and serious attacks which, he judged, were caused by some form of unconscious imitation. It seemed to him essential that patients who were liable to suffer from these attacks should be segregated, as far as possible, and if the available funds allowed, from other patients who might act as their 'models'. In this, and in stressing the importance of the early diagnosis and prompt treatment of hysterical patients, Charcot made one of the greatest of his contributions to his chosen branch of medical science. Hardly less important was his insistence on the fact that men as well as women were liable to suffer from hysterical conditions, and that the age-old association of hysteria with abnormal movements of the uterus had no foundation in fact. His opinion came to carry great weight in courts of law where 'millions of dollars' – to use Charcot's own phrase – might change hands, one way or the other, in disputed cases where heavy damages were being sought. Frequently, he asserted, the victim of an accident might be rendered, by hysteria, incapable of any form of movement for months or even years, though he, or she, would have appeared to have sustained little or no discernible physical injury. Charcot's view helped to clear many unfortunates from unjust charges of malingering. As Sigmund Freud was to write, later, of Charcot's work in the observation of the neuroses:

> He began to turn his attention almost exclusively to hysteria, thus suddenly focussing general attention on this subject. This most enigmatic of all nervous diseases – no workable point of view having yet been found from which physicians could regard it – had just at this time come very much into discredit, and this ill-repute related not only to the patients but was extended to the physicians who treated this neurosis. The general opinion was that anything might happen in hysteria; hysterics found no credit whatsoever. First of all Charcot's work restored dignity to the subject; gradually the sneering attitude, which the hysteric could reckon on meeting when she told her story, was given up; she was no longer a malingerer, since Charcot had thrown the whole weight of his authority on the side of the reality and objectivity of hysteria, thus suddenly focusing general attention on this scale the act of liberation commemorated in the picture of Pinel which adorned the lecture hall of the Salpêtrière.[8]

As Charcot's successes in dealing with hysterical patients became widely publicised, sufferers travelled – or were taken – to him from many different parts of the world. One such – a clever and industrious boy who was being brought up in South Russia – suddenly started to suffer from severe headaches. The local doctors, presuming that the boy was developing a brain tumour, were far from optimistic, but the boy's father, who was exceedingly fond of his son, decided to take him to France to consult Charcot. Charcot, in one of his lectures to his students, described the case:

> From the very first interview, we were able to give him

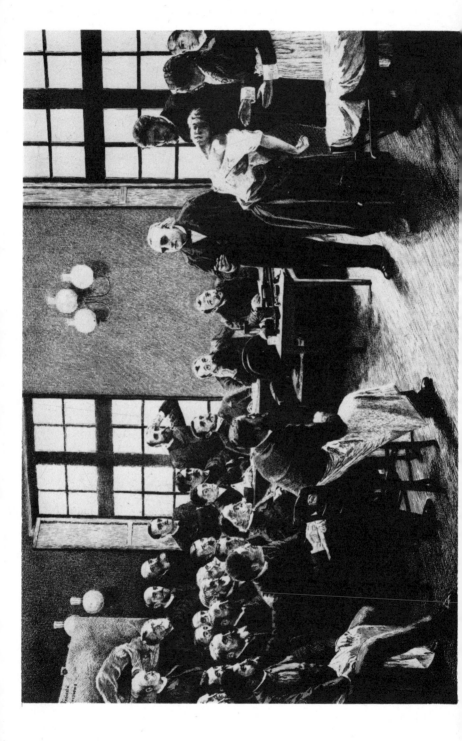

hope. Not only will the child live, but we can affirm without hesitation that the child will make a complete recovery. The headache was in the habit of returning every evening about 5 p.m. followed shortly afterwards by convulsive attacks. The occurrence of the attack at the same time of day for five months offers a strong presumption of hysteria.[9]

It was interesting, went on Charcot, to watch, each day, the father's behaviour at the expected time of attack:

He takes out his watch and questions his son and asks if he is suffering. If the reply is 'yes' he displays an amount of solicitude which is respectable, no doubt, but which certainly tends to foster the patient's condition and to maintain the regularity of his symptoms.[10]

Charcot, feeling sure of his diagnosis, and judging shrewdly that the father's anxieties were helping to perpetuate the boy's excitable nervous condition, tried to isolate the child from his desperately worried parent. The father, however, would not agree to be separated from his son, and every day at the same hour he would wait expectantly for the boy to be overtaken by another attack. The boy, of course, would 'oblige' in the usual way, and this went on until Charcot decided that the boy would have to be moved away to a sanatorium. Even then, the father tried to haunt the approaches to the building so that he could ask everyone who left the place if they knew how his son was faring. At last, Charcot was driven to insist that the father should keep right away from the sanatorium and that he should have no contact at all with anyone who worked there. Within a month, the boy from South Russia was completely cured and could be safely discharged.

Charcot's preoccupation with hysteria did not prevent him from carrying out, with his assistants, much valuable research into other nervous disorders. While Koch and

Pasteur were demonstrating the infective nature of so many human diseases, Charcot and his closest colleagues were managing to show positively that not a few of their patients were suffering from neurological conditions that had some constitutional origin and were in no way due to harmful organisms that entered the patient's bodies from the environment, to over-consumption of alcohol, or to any other comparable cause. By the end of the nineteenth century, thanks largely to Charcot, most of the neurologic diseases known today had been accurately identified and, in the words of Georges Guillain, a later occupant of Charcot's professional chair, 'had been exquisitely correlated with their anatomic and pathologic substrata'.[11]

Axel Munthe, who was one of the most articulate men ever to work at the Salpêtrière, described, some years after he was asked to leave the place, some of Charcot's more sensational experiments in the field of hypnotism.

The credit for having discovered hypnotic techniques –as far as Europe goes – is generally given to Franz Anton Mesmer (1734–1815). Mesmer was an Austrian physician who was working in France at the time of the Revolution. At Mesmer's sensational séances, his patients would normally be asked to sit round an open tub from which magnetised metal rods would protrude. Some of the patients would then develop some sort of crisis or fit, after which they would wake up either cured or greatly improved. Mesmer found, later, that he could dispense with the magnetised rods. It was sufficient, it seemed, for him just to touch a patient or even to put the tip of one of his fingers into water before the patient drank it. He concluded that he had been endowed with some kind of 'animal magnetism', which he could store in his body and pass on to others whom he might wish to heal. His ideas were discredited by the members of a commission set up officially to investigate his claims, and he was widely regarded, then, as a 'quack'. But a belief in the possible uses of his 'mesmeric' process lingered on in some quarters, nevertheless.

By 1840, several physicians such as a Doctor John Elliotson of London and a Doctor James Esdaile in Calcutta were putting many of their patients into hypnotic trances, finding that in this condition the patients could undergo major surgical operations – even, occasionally, leg amputations – without appearing to suffer much pain. Doctor Elliotson was a firm believer in the efficacy of Mesmer's invisible 'animal magnetism', and he was also a powerful advocate of the metal nickel which, he said, was particularly valuable for the induction of trances. The Editor of *The Lancet* medical journal surreptitiously substituted lead for zinc before Elliotson carried out some of his experiments. As the lead appeared to be just as effective as the doctor had said that nickel would be, the *Lancet* editor denounced the doctor's teachings as 'mesmeric humbug'.

It was a Manchester surgeon, James Braid (1795–1860), who must be regarded as the founding father of modern hypnotism. Watching some public demonstration of 'mesmeric treatment' given by a Swiss magnetizer named Lafontaine, whom he believed to be an impostor, Braid was profoundly moved, in spite of his scepticism, by the powerful influence that Lafontaine appeared to be exerting on his patients. Not believing that 'magnetism' of any kind was flowing out of Lafontaine, Braid coined a quite new word – suggested, it seems, by the Greek word *hypnos,* meaning 'sleep' – to denote the process by which a patient can be put into a sleep-like trance. His discovery that hypnosis could often be induced by persuading a patient to gaze fixedly at some stationary or slowly oscillating object was to have a profound influence, later, on those who were studying the subject under J.-M. Charcot at the Salpêtrière.

Charcot's interest in Braid's techniques led to the French doctor carrying out, from the year 1878, research on the use of hypnotism with hysterical patients. He was ready to try almost any new therapeutic process, however bizarre, for he had recently been experimenting at the Salpêtrière with some metallotherapic techniques developed by a Doctor Victor

Burq. Burq had claimed that he could restore feeling and movement to the insensible limbs of hysterical patients by putting plaques made of gold and other metals on to the parts of the patients that were paralysed – and Charcot had found that Burq's methods did bring, in many instances, almost instantaneous relief.

Following Braid, then, Charcot managed to send a number of his patients into hypnotic trances by concentrating their attention on prescribed objects until they were overcome by fatigue. He succeeded, in other cases, by putting gentle pressure on his patients' eyeballs; by exposing the patients to bright lights; or by exposing the patients to the sounds of loud blows on a gong. Once a patient had passed into a cataleptic state, easily recognizable because the patient's pulse would slacken and his or her breathing would become appreciably lighter, Charcot would demonstrate to his students and, sometimes, to members of the general public, that his patient had become totally unaware of his or her surroundings, and that part at least of the patient's body had become insensitive to pain. Two pins, for testing anaesthesia, were kept conspicuously in a pincushion on Charcot's desk. When he had his patients under hypnotism, Charcot thought, he would be able to study more carefully any constitutional tendencies towards hysteria they might have inherited because these would be shown in an exaggerated form.

The work being done by Charcot on hypnotism at the Salpêtrière was brought dramatically to the attention of a very wide public by a violent controversy that arose between Charcot, with his Parisian associates, and an obscure country physician called Ambroise-Auguste Liébault who lived and practised at Nancy. Nancy is not far from Strasbourg, where much work was being done on mesmeric techniques by the members of a local 'Society of Harmony', and it is possible that Liébault's interests were aroused and his latent talents discovered by his enthusiastic neighbours. Having apparently cured several of his patients by suggestion while they were in hypnotic trances, Liébault gave up orthodox medical practice and started to run a free clinic, based on hypnotism, using a shed in his garden as a centre. Liébault was a very successful operator in his chosen field, being able to hypnotise nine out of every ten of his patients with surprising rapidity, but his reputation remained a purely local one until, in 1882, he managed to cure the apparently chronic sciatica of one of the patients of Hippolyte Bernheim, who was Professor of Medicine at Strasbourg University. At first, Bernheim was sceptical of Liébault's powers, but after watching the Nancy man at work in his clinic he was completely converted, and after that tried to hypnotise as many as he could of the patients who came to his own clinic.

The conflict between the Parisians and the members of the circle at Nancy and Strasbourg began when Bernheim, in 1884, started to publish his ideas about hypnotism. The phenomenon involved no physical forces and no physiological processes, he postulated, but was, instead, entirely psychological. Liébault, independently of Bernheim, let people know of some experiments he had been carrying out with 'mesmerised' and 'unmesmerised' spring water. Having found that he could carry out 'cures' just as successfully with the latter as with the former, he announced that he was pinning his faith, thereafter, in the powers of suggestion. Charcot and his friends in Paris, who were still working away enthusiastically with their magnets and metal plaques, were not impressed by Bernheim's and Liébault's views and said so publicly. Medical commentators suggest, now, that the Salpêtrians' metallic devices may have fulfilled very much the same faith-healing purpose as Liébault's fresh pure water.

The differences between the men in the Salpêtrière and the members of the 'School of Nancy' brought to the notice of thousands of members of the lay public the dramatic results that could be achieved with the hypnotic process if it were used by the unscrupulous for improper purposes. Almost at once, perfectly innocent medical men who had a readiness to experiment and honourable and upright members of provincial Societies of Harmony started to appear in the docks of criminal courts and were accused there of seducing or raping their more attractive patients while those patients were under the influence of hypnotism. In other cases, people accused of murder, robbery and other crimes claimed that they had been forced by some hypnotist to do what they would never have wanted to do if they had been in their rightful minds. In England, a doctor named Kingsbury was accused of persuading one of his lady patients, when under hypnosis, to make a will under which he would inherit a fortune. For more than a decade, the intriguing possibilities open to dishonest hypnotists made a favourite topic of conversation at fashionable dinner tables.

Until he died of heart trouble in 1893, J.-M. Charcot remained one of France's most commanding and influential figures, being on the friendliest of terms with Louis Pasteur, Daniel Hack Tuke, and other great innovators who were striving to improve the human condition. He is remembered now with particular respect because Sigmund Freud, in 1885, obtained a lectureship in neuropathology at the University of Vienna, and then, assisted by a travelling fellowship, went to Paris where he spent a full year, studying in detail all the relevant researches that were being carried out at the Salpêtrière. Although Freud was to use Charcot's hypnotic techniques for only a comparatively short time after he returned to Vienna (he was interested, primarily, in helping his most neurotic patients to recall disturbing events and he soon developed his own system of psychoanalysis which he found more effective for this) he was happy to pay tribute to the pioneering role that Charcot had played in the continuing exploration of the unconscious mind:

He [Charcot] was heard to say that the greatest satisfaction a man can experience is to see something new, that is, to recognize it as new, and he constantly returned with repeated observations to the subject of the difficulties and the value of such 'seeing'. He wondered how it happened that in the practice of medicine men could only see what they had already been taught to see; he described how wonderful it was suddenly to see new things – new diseases – though they were probably as old as the human race; he said that he often had to admit that he could now see many a thing which for thirty years in his wards he had ignored.[12]

No physician, continued Freud, would need to be reminded of the wealth of new outlines which the science of neuro-pathology had gained through Charcot's efforts, or of the much greater keenness and accuracy that had been made possible by the aid of his observations.

# 14

## Alternative Medicine
## in the Nineteenth Century

*Man is a creature who lives not upon bread alone but
principally by catchwords.*

ROBERT LOUIS STEVENSON, 1850–94

At the beginning of the nineteenth century, quack doctors
and other unqualified practitioners of medicine and 'surgery'
were as active and as respected as ever.

Most numerous were the herbalists. These were more or
less direct descendants of the men and women who, in earlier
years, had been practising the simplest forms of 'folk
medicine', usually under the influence of Nicholas Culpe-
per, author of the *Physical Directory* published in London in
1649. Mrs. Gaskell, in her novel *Mary Barton*, published in
1848, sketched in words one of these modest healers:

> She had been out all day in the fields, gathering wild herbs
> for drinks and medicine, for in addition to her invaluable
> qualities as a sick nurse and her worldly occupation as a
> washerwoman, she added a considerable knowledge of
> hedge and field simples; and on fine days, when no more
> profitable occupation offered itself, she used to ramble off
> into the lanes and meadows as far as her legs could carry
> her. This evening she had returned loaded with nettles,
> and her first object was to light a candle and see to hang
> them up in bunches in every available place in her cellar
> room . . . The cellar window was oddly festooned with all
> manner of hedgerow, ditch and field plants, which we are
> accustomed to call valueless, but which have a powerful
> effect either for good or for evil, and consequently much

used among the poor. The room was strewed, hung, and darkened with these bunches, which emitted no very fragrant odour in their process of drying.

As late as 1831, 'genuine and authentic accounts' were being published of the Life and Memoirs of 'that surprising and wonderful man Henry Jenkins, commonly called Old Jenkins, of Ellerton upon Swale in Yorkshire, who lived to the amazing age of one hundred and sixty-nine years and upwards, which is seventeen years longer than Old Parr, and the oldest man to be met with in the annals of England'. Jenkins, who died in 1670, had been a collector of 'valuable recipes', the greater part of which he had given to an Hon. Mrs. Ann Saville, who had written them down so that they could be circulated more widely. The disappointments suffered by those who, over a century and a half, relied on Jenkins' recommendations must have been tragic. For 'A Windy Rupture', for instance, he prescribed

> Warm cow-dung well, spread it thick on leather, strew some cummin[1] seeds on it, and apply it hot; when it is cold, put on a fresh one, and keep the child in bed for two days.

'A Cancer in the Breast' inspired Jenkins (or the Hon. Mrs. Saville) to this:

> An inveterate bleeding cancer, of twenty years standing, was perfectly cured by only drinking, twice a day, of the juice of clider, or goosegrass, a quarter of a pint, and applying the bruised leaves as a poultice to the affected parts. – Or, boil gently the juice of clider in fresh hog's lard, (equal parts), and apply it night and morning, as a plaster, to the part affected. – Or, if not broke, rub the whole breast, morning and evening, with spirits of hartshorn, sweet oil, and laudanum, equal parts. – Or, apply celandine and goose dung, beat well together, and spread on a fine linen rag, morning and evening, this will both cleanse and heal the sores.

The popularity of herbalism in Britain and other European countries was stimulated, early in the nineteenth century, by some new thinking from the United States of America. The chief innovator there was one Samuel Thomson. Thomson was born in 1769, the son of an impoverished New Hampshire farmer, and had little formal education. Having no liking for ordinary farm work he preferred, when he was young, to spend most of his time wandering about the fields and woods near his home, studying the herbs that he found there and investigating their medicinal properties. He took a particular interest in the plant known as *lobelia inflata*, the crushed seeds of which, he found, would induce perspiration and vomiting. When he was twenty-one, Thomson was compelled to take over the management of the family farm, but he soon lost interest in this, preferring, in his own words, 'to make use of the gift which nature or the God of nature has implanted in me.' Working from the assumption that all human diseases are produced by cold, and that any medicine which helps to generate internal heat will help to hasten a patient's recovery, Thomson set out to make the advantages of *lobelia inflata* – and, to a lesser extent, other herbal remedies – nationally known. Soon he was the proprietor of a busy drug shop in Boston, Massachusetts, and the overseer of a chain of agencies spread widely over America. The publication of two books by Thomson – his *New Guide to Health* or *The Botanic Family Physician* (1822) and *Learned Quackery Exposed* (1824) – made his reputation throughout his native Continent.

Thomson's ideas, known generally as the 'Thomsonian System', were carried over the Atlantic by a vigorous American herbalist who called himself Doctor Coffin. When he started his mission in London in 1838, Doctor Coffin gave out that he had been taught the value of herbs by an old Indian woman who had cured him of tuberculosis by traditional herbal remedies. Not many people in the English capital took a real interest in the American's teachings, however, and soon 'Doctor Coffin' moved away to the less sophisticated cities and towns of north-east England, where his lectures were given more attention. From Leeds, in 1845, he published a short treatise that he called his *Botanic Guide to Health*. In his preface to this booklet, the American claimed that a knowledge of nature was not necessarily compatible with college life. This knowledge had to be sought for in the woods and forests, he asserted, where 'each sun-lit vale or verdant meadow contains some agent of a remedial kind'. The millions who bought copies of his treatise would be able to prescribe successfully for themselves, the herbalist went on.

While Samuel Thomson, in America, was formulating his Botanic System, Charles Gottfried Samuel Hahnemann, in Europe, was creating homoeopathy.

Born in 1775, Hahnemann had the degree of Doctor of Medicine conferred on him in 1799 by the University of Erlangen. He practised for a time, in a variety of places, but he became increasingly dissatisfied with the orthodox medical techniques of the time and he found it difficult to make a respectable living. At last, in the first year of his married life, he gave up medical practice altogether and tried to support his wife and child by chemistry, a subject in which he had had little or no tuition, and by writing and translating scientific books.

Hahnemann started to develop the ideas with which he is now chiefly associated while he was translating into German the second edition of the *Materia Medica* that had been compiled by William Cullen, the original instructor of William Hunter. Cullen, Hahnemann noticed, had written that cinchona, or 'Peruvian Bark', was used with great effect in the treatment of malaria. He had added that the drug's beneficient effects were due to its tonic action on the stomach of the patient. This was too much for Hahnemann to accept, and he added a lengthy objection. If strong bitters and strong astringents were combined, he pointed out, a compound would be produced that would have an even greater tonic effect than cinchona. But, he went on, in all Eternity no fever specific could ever be made from a compound of this kind, and he thought that Cullen should have accounted for this.

Next, Hahnemann described some of the experiments that he himself had been carrying out with cinchona. Daily for several days, he wrote, he had been taking four drams of the drug. Each time he had repeated the dose, his feet and finger tips had become cold, and other symptoms had followed which were typical of malaria. Each time he had stopped taking the cinchona, he had returned rapidly to a state of good health.

In the next three years, Hahnemann spent much of his time in trying the effects of various drugs on himself. Then he published in a medical paper a short article called *A New Principle for Ascertaining the Curative Properties of Drugs, and some Examinations of the Previous Principles*. In this essay, Hahnemann suggested that a doctor should use only those remedies which would have the power to create, in a healthy body, symptoms similar to those that might be seen in the sick person being treated. This directive became known as 'The Law of Similars'. If a drug of a 'contrary' type were administered to a patient for any prolonged period of time, he concluded, the condition of that patient would almost inevitably worsen.

Next, Hahnemann announced that he had found by experiment that if the dosage of a drug were gradually but steadily reduced, the power of that drug to cure would actually be increased. This led him to try the technical expedient of reducing the dosage of a drug in carefully regulated stages until the patient for whom the drug had been prescribed was actually receiving a microscopic dose, when, Hahnemann claimed, the drug was more effective than ever before. This method, known today by homoeopathists as 'serial dilution', was immediately ridiculed by most of the more orthodox medical men who heard about it.

To counter this opposition, Hahnemann set up an 'Institute of Homoeopathy' in his own home. He advertised in the Press tutorial courses that would last for six months, and which all properly qualified medical men were invited to attend. His plan failed utterly. The advertisements did not produce a single applicant. So Hahnemann next managed to get himself appointed, early in 1812, to a professorial chair at the University of Leipzig. He was careful to keep very quiet about his homoeopathic beliefs while he was undergoing the process of selection, but once he had started to lecture he made his purposes clear: he was at the University principally to expound the advantages of homoeopathy to anyone who would be prepared to listen to him. He can hardly be said to have set about achieving his objectives in a rational way, for he chose to appear in the lecture hall in grotesque and comical costumes, and he delivered his material, much of which consisted of strident abuse of orthodox medical practitioners, in a melodramatic and sometimes even hysterical manner. His students soon dwindled in numbers.

The first signs that homoeopathy might become a respected medical technique came during the serious typhus epidemic that followed the retreat of Napoleon's armies from Moscow. Because, under Hahnemann's methods, relatively small doses of 'curative' drugs were administered, a number of his patients survived, and his reputation started to improve. This provoked a violent reaction from the professional apothecaries, who saw clearly that if Hahnemann's disciples were allowed to practise under the Master's principles, their own livelihoods would be seriously threatened. So in February 1820, before the Council of the Town of Leipzig, they accused Hahnemann of infringing their traditional rights and privileges. In vain, Hahnemann pleaded that homoeopathic remedies were prescribed only for the patients of recognised homoeopathists, and that no true homoeopathist would wish to make money by prescribing and selling his remedies to anybody else. The members of the Council listened politely to Hahnemann, but they ordered him to stop distributing his own medicines or face a crippling fine.

Unfortunately for the apothecaries, Hahnemann happened at the time to be treating a very influential patient – the intemperate Prince Schwarzenberg of Austria, who was a cousin of the King of Saxony. Afraid that he might have to do without Hahnemann's aid, the Prince appealed to the King, telling his cousin that since he had been relying on Doctor Hahnemann's remedies his 'attacks' had been less severe. The King announced that no further harassment of Doctor Hahnemann would be allowed. Hahnemann's relief was only temporary, however, for soon after that the Prince started to drink heavily again and in his weakened state allowed some 'orthodox' medical men to bleed him. Hahnemann arrived just as the operation he despised was taking place. The homoeopathist, bitterly offended, withdrew at once and refused to return. Five weeks later, the Prince died. An autopsy was conducted by a team of doctors headed by a Doctor Clarus, who was one of Hahnemann's most malevolent enemies. At the end of the examination, Clarus drafted and signed a report in which he placed the blame for the royal drunkard's death firmly on Hahnemann's shoulders. The Government of Saxony were convinced by this pronouncement of the evils of homoeopathy and passed a decree which would prevent anyone except an authorised apothecary from dispensing any medicine.[2] Hahnemann had had enough. With few apparent regrets he left the hostile atmosphere of Saxony and went to live in Anhalt-Coethen, where, he had been assured by the reigning Duke, he and his assistants would be allowed to practise freely and publish more or less what they liked.

In Anhalt-Coethen, Hahnemann lived and worked for more than ten years. During that time, he was able to convince physicians in many other parts of the world of the effectiveness of his methods. Doctors in America were particularly quick to try homoeopathic techniques, news of Hahnemann's methods having been taken there in 1825 by a Doctor Gram, of Boston, Massachusetts, who had been studying in Copenhagen. In 1833, an Academy for teaching homoeopathic methods was founded at Allentown, near Philadelphia, and three years later the influential Hahnemann Medical College was founded in Philadelphia itself.

Homoeopathy is still practised in a few places today.

The support given by the Duke of Anhalt-Coethen to Charles Hahnemann was typical of the aristocratic patronage sought at the time by many on the fringes of 'real' medicine. The purveyors of the 'patent' and 'proprietary' medicines popular throughout the nineteenth century were never slow to seek such patronage. On Saturday 29 October 1836 this advertisement appeared in *The Times*:

> Her Serene Highness the Landgravine of Hesse Homburg; the Dukes of Devonshire, Beaufort, Rutland, Sutherland, and Buccleuch; the Marquises of Lansdowne, Winchester, Abercorn, Ailesbury, Tavistock, and Blandford; the Earls of Errol, Harrowby, Eldon, Minto, and Amherst; the Viscounts Melbourne, Palmerston, and Howick; the Lords Plunket, Hill, Murray, and numerous other distinguished personages, have given their unqualified approbation to the FAMILY ANTIBILIOUS PILLS prepared by Mr. COCKLE, Apothecary Extraordinary to Her Serene Highness. These pills may be had of any respectable medicine vender.

Below it was this:

> CHING'S WORM LOZENGES are patronised by the first noblemen in the kingdom, as well as by the following Honourable Ladies, who have given this medicine to their own children, and also to the poor of their respective neighbourhoods, with unparalleled success: – Her Grace the Duchess of Leeds, her Grace the Duchess of Rutland, the Right Hon. the Countess of Darnley, the Right Hon. Lady Caroline Capel, the Right Hon. Lady Elizabeth Spencer, the Hon. Lady Boston, the Hon. Lady Say and Sele, the Right Hon. the Countess of Shaftesbury, the Right Hon. the Countess of Mountnorris, the Right Hon. the Countess of Cork, the Right Hon. Lady Lucy Bridgeman, Lady Page Turner, Lady Lovet, and many

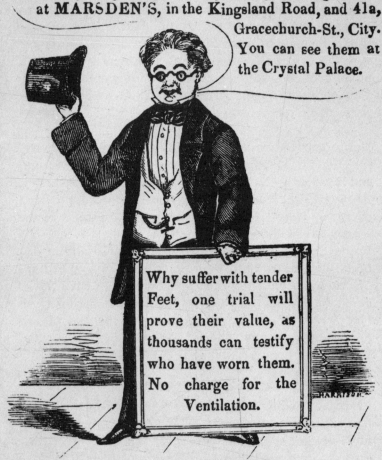

A handbill for ventilated boots

other ladies of the first rank and character. It is a fact established by the annual bills of mortality, that one half of the children born are cut off before attaining seven years of age, and the fruitful source of this mortality is found to exist in that foul state of the stomach and bowels which produces the generation of worms. As the safe restorer of infantine health, in this critical state, CHING'S WORM LOZENGES have long held a distinguished reputation. As an opening medicine in spring and summer, and for foulness of the stomach and bowels, and convulsions, although worms may not exist, it is allowed to be superior to any other. The genuine will have on the Government stamp 'Evan Edwards, 67, St. Paul's'. In packets, 1s. 1½d. and boxes at 2s. 9d. each. Sold also by Stradling, Royal Exchange-gates, Cornhill.

One of the most successful of all the nineteenth century 'venders' of patent and proprietary medicines was Thomas Holloway.

Holloway was born at Devonport – then called 'Plymouth Dock' – on 22 September 1800. His father had been a warrant officer in a militia regiment. When he retired from the service, Holloway Senior had entered the bakery trade, and at the time of his decease was running a grocery and bakery shop in the market place at Penzance. After his father's death, young Thomas worked for a time with his mother and his brother Henry in the shop. Then, finding the scope for enterprise in Penzance rather limited, he departed for London. By 1836, he was operating as a general merchant and foreign commercial agent from a suite of offices at 13 Broad Street Buildings.

To Holloway's office came, one day, an Italian trader called Felix Albinola. Albinola had been born in Turin. From there he had moved to London where he made a sparse living by selling leeches to medical men. As a side line, Albinola carried an ointment that he called 'Albinola's', or the 'St. Come et St. Damien' ointment. Holloway offered to introduce Albinola to the authorities of St. Thomas's Hospital, in the hope that they would give the Italian testimonials that vouched for the usefulness and value of his ointment. When they did so, Holloway must have wondered if a similar ointment, recommended in much the same way by influential medical authorities, and widely advertised, might not provide an agreeable source of income for himself.

According to Holloway's own account, the news that 'Holloway's Family Ointment' was on sale was first made public on 15 October 1837. The earliest surviving advertisement for the ointment appeared in *The Town* of 16 June 1838. In this advertisement, the curative value of Holloway's Ointment was vouched for by 'Herbert Mayo, Senior Surgeon, Middlesex Hospital'. Doctor Mayo became, later, President of the Royal College of Physicians. The advertisement must have provoked a passionate reaction from the Italian, for an announcement in a later issue of *The Town* warned all members of the public that Doctor Mayo's letter of recommendation had been written in respect of Albinola's Ointment, the composition of which had never been revealed. Signor Albinola's defence of his own preparation cannot have done him much good, however, for in the following year he was committed to a debtors' prison, after which nothing whatsoever was heard of him.

Having beaten his rival from the field, Holloway took a large building in The Strand, referring to this place as his 'Patent Medicine Warehouse'. He started to spend every penny he could spare – and some that he could not – on advertising, in a variety of ways, his ointment and the 'Holloway's Pills' he had also decided to produce. At least once each day he would go to the Thames-side docks so that he personally could bring his preparations to the notice of the Captains of the vessels and their passengers, who would shortly be sailing to the most distant parts of the world. For a time his efforts met with little success and, falling into serious financial difficulties, he was forced to compound with his creditors, several of whom were newspaper proprietors.

Then the tide started to turn, as steadily increasing

numbers of people began to buy Holloway's preparations. In 1842, Holloway spent £5000 on advertising; in 1845, £10,000; in 1851, £20,000; in 1864, £40,000; and in 1882 £45,000. Directions for the use of his pills and ointment were translated into nearly every known tongue, including Arabic, Armenian, Chinese, Turkish and most of the vernaculars of India, and his advertisements were to be found in the newspapers of every civilized country.

As Holloway's fame and private fortune grew he had to contend with a number of misfortunes. In 1850, for instance, he was disturbed to see that his brother Henry had started to sell some so-called 'Holloway's Pills and Ointment' from an address not far from his own warehouse in The Strand, and he was forced to obtain an injunction that would compel Henry to cease doing this. In 1860 he took a Doctor Sillon into his employment and commissioned him to introduce the 'genuine' Holloway wares into France, but the laws of that country were not framed in a way that favoured the purveyors of secret remedies, and the project had to be dropped, a decision of Holloway's which resulted in further litigation. In 1867, Holloway was compelled to vacate his warehouse in The Strand because it was built on land needed for the construction of the new Royal Courts of Justice, so he removed to New Oxford Street. There he was able to increase his staff until he was employing – without counting outdoor staff and part-time assistants – over a hundred people.

In spite of Thomas Holloway's great wealth – the profits of his business reached at least £50,000 per year, and he added considerably to this by judicious investment in stocks and shares – the Patent Medicine King lived on a relatively modest scale. At first he lived in premises attached to his successive London warehouses. Later, he lived in a country house at Tittenhurst, near Sunninghill in Berkshire. As he grew old, he tried to dispose of much of his personal fortune. Efforts that he made to use some of his money for the benefit of the people of his native town were frustrated by the local authorities, who did not think that they should approve officially of the sale of patent medicines. Advised, eventually, by the philanthropist Lord Shaftesbury, Holloway decided to build and equip at Virginia Water a Sanatorium that would serve as a sanctuary for mentally afflicted members of the lower middle classes. This large building, containing nearly five hundred rooms and capable of accommodating two hundred and forty-five patients, was opened on 15 June 1885 by Their Royal Highnesses the Prince and Princess of Wales. Meanwhile, Holloway had bought ninety acres of land on Egham Hill on which he proposed to found a College for Ladies. This institution, which could accommodate two hundred and fifty students, was opened by Queen Victoria in 1886. Flamboyantly designed, and still housing Holloway's valuable collection of paintings, the Royal Holloway College is now one of the most remarkable assets of the University of London.

The value of extensive and persistent advertising, realised so profitably by Thomas Holloway, was also appreciated by his contemporary Thomas Beecham. Beecham was born at Witney, in Oxfordshire, on 3 December 1820. When he was about twenty-five years old he opened a chemist's shop at Wigan in Lancashire and there, inspired probably by advertisements for Holloway's pills, he concocted a formula for the manufacture of 'Beecham's Pills', his first patent medicine licence being issued at Liverpool and dated 8 July 1847.

In 1859, Beecham moved his business to the new town of St. Helens, which was midway between Wigan and Liverpool. It was to be a fortunate move. Shortly after he started work at St. Helens, Beecham happened to hear an appreciative remark made by a woman who had just purchased some of his pills. 'They are worth a guinea a box!' she said. A guinea being quite a large sum of money in the England of those days, the remark caught Thomas Beecham's fancy and thereafter he made the slogan 'Worth a Guinea a Box!' the advertising motto of his little concern.

From then on the Beecham business started to prosper and

its rate of achievement accelerated even more after 1866, when Thomas Beecham's elder son Joseph joined the firm, bringing to it much youthful energy and an unusually enterprising outlook. By 1885, Joseph felt able to encourage his father to build at a considerable cost a new factory at St. Helens. From St. Helens, the work of the Beechams spread to New York, where Joseph established a second factory that would act as a base for the family's transatlantic trade. By the end of the nineteenth century, there were 'Beechams' Pills' factories or agencies in a number of other countries, and the slogan 'Worth a Guinea a Box!' was known virtually all over the world, inducing millions of people – even those who had no idea what a 'guinea' was – to buy the Beechams' pills. And well into the present century, in Christian countries school children could be heard chanting rudely:

Hark the Herald Angels sing:
'Beechams' Pills are just the thing!'

When Samuel Thomson's disciple 'Doctor Coffin' moved from London to the north of England and published his *Botanic Guide to Health*, as described earlier in this chapter, a London herbalist called John Skelton felt compelled to leave his metropolitan practice so that he could support Coffin in the remote provinces. Skelton, speaking familiar English, was even more influential among the working class members of the crowded Northern manufacturing towns than Coffin had been, and he spent the two years 1849 and 1850 in lecturing and in engaging agents who would buy Coffin's herbs and who would then practise as 'medical botanists'.

At one of Skelton's meetings, held at Nottingham, an earnest young man called John Boot was present. Boot had inherited from his mother, who was a profoundly religious woman, a single-minded intention to devote his life to the service of mankind, and as she had been intensely interested in herbs and folk medicines he listened to Skelton's teachings with enthusiasm. 'Medical botany is an eternal truth, and its reception by mankind can only be in proportion to the zeal, talents, faith, industry and application of the means necessary to command it', thundered Skelton. Boot reacted to this challenge with evangelistic fervour and before long he opened a little shop in Goosegate on the northern edge of the town. From this shop, which he called 'The British and American Botanic Establishment', Boot sold 'vegetable remedies' both wholesale and retail. He held consultations in the little parlour at the back of his shop, and before five years had elapsed he was able to claim confidently that with his herbal medicaments he had successfully treated almost every kind of disease.

Soon the members of the medical profession, alarmed by the popularity of 'Coffin', Skelton, Boot and other herbal healers, attempted to persuade the members of the British parliament to pass a Medical Reform Bill which would prevent men who were not properly qualified from practising at all. The herbalists countered this by setting up a 'National Medical Reform League' and John Boot was one of the League's principal advocates in the Nottingham area. In spite of his insistence on the effectiveness of herbal remedies, however, John Boot's health broke down while he was still a comparatively young man, and his little business had to be carried on, after he died at the early age of forty-four, by his still younger widow, who had depending on her a son named Jesse, who was then aged ten, and a daughter Jane who was less than two years old.

As soon as Jesse was old enough to leave school, he joined his mother in the work of the shop, tramping many miles each week to collect herbs and helping her in the business of preparing potions and pills. By the time he was in his teens, Jesse Boot had learned practically everything that his mother could teach him and he had started to take over the management of the enterprise. By this time, though, young Boot had begun to realise that believers in medical botany were not increasing in numbers as rapidly as his father and mother had hoped. There seemed, in fact, to be fewer and fewer each year. So he started to add the more popular patent medicines to his stock, explaining, years later, his ideas:

> After all, there was nothing at all remarkable about my methods. They were simply the application of common sense. I found that everywhere articles, especially drugs, were being sold at ridiculously high prices, and were sold without any regard to neatness and attractiveness. My idea was simply to buy tons where others bought hundredweights or pounds, thus buying much more cheaply, and making all the articles I sold look as attractive as possible. I made, too, as I could afford to make, a substantial reduction to customers who bought a quantity. Thus I sold bicarbonate of potash at a penny an ounce, but I only charged sevenpence for a pound, and sixpence a pound (less than a halfpenny an ounce) for larger quantities. On patent medicines, too, I found that I could knock off twopence or so, and still make a nice little profit.[3]

The success of Jesse Boot's commonsense methods bordered on the sensational. By the end of the nineteenth century, 'Boots Cash Chemists' shops were in full operation in Bath, Bedford, Bristol, Cambridge, Coventry, Kettering, Lowestoft, Luton, Manchester, Norwich, Peterborough, Stafford, Swansea, Walsall, Wednesbury, Wellingborough, and many other towns. Before Boot, totally crippled with rheumatoid arthritis, finally relinquished day-to-day control of his group of companies in 1920, he and his wife were able to claim, with confidence, that he had built up by his own energetic enterprise the largest firm of chemists in the world.

# X-Rays and their Application

... 'It is,' says Chadband, 'the ray of rays, the sun of
suns, the moon of moons, the star of stars.
It is the light of Terewth . . .'

CHARLES DICKENS, *Bleak House*

William Conrad Röntgen, who was to be one of the most
dedicated researchers of the nineteenth century, was born on
27 March 1845 at Lennep, in pleasant country near the
industrial cities of the Ruhr valley. The place is now known
as Remscheid, and it is in West Germany. In May 1848 the
Röntgen family moved to Apeldoorn in Holland. Within a
few months, they had become Dutch citizens.

William Conrad received his early education in the primary
and secondary public schools at Apeldoorn. In December
1862 he entered the Technical School at Utrecht. There he
took courses in algebra, chemistry, geometry, physics and
technology. He was a lively student who enjoyed making
ingenious gadgets. His educational progress suffered a severe
setback when he was unjustly accused of executing, on a
blackboard, an unkind caricature of his principal teacher.
After refusing to reveal the true identity of the 'artist',
Röntgen was summarily dismissed from the school. Finding
that this would prevent him from becoming an orthodox
university student, he joined the mechanical technical division of the Zurich Polytechnic.

Most of the credit for Röntgen's rise to eminence as a
physicist must be given to August Kundt who, in 1868, took
the Chair of Physics at the Polytechnic. After graduating
from the school in engineering, Röntgen stayed on to take a
further course, in mathematics, and to attend Kundt's
lectures on the theory of light. Working in Kundt's laboratory and helping Kundt to reorganise it, Röntgen learned

to be exceedingly meticulous, and he also learned how to make the best possible use of equipment that was, by the standards of the time, no more than merely adequate. It was here that he undertook his earliest physical experiments on the varying properties of gases, and while he was engaged on these he gradually came to realise that this was the kind of work to which he was best suited. After a year spent in close association with Kundt, Röntgen submitted a thesis on gases to the University of Zurich and on the basis of this he was awarded, on 22 June 1869, a Doctorate of Philosophy.

Although relations between Kundt and Röntgen were occasionally stormy – as, for example, when Kundt found Röntgen using some especially delicate instruments which Kundt had been carefully reserving for his own use – the older man asked Röntgen to accompany him as his first assistant when, in 1870, Kundt was offered and accepted the Chair of Physics at the University of Würzburg. Once again, in the old university buildings on the Neubaustrasse in Würzburg, Röntgen found that he would be compelled to work in a poorly equipped department, commenting, a little sourly, 'A real physicist must build a laboratory with a test glass and a cigar box'. Kundt countered this by suggesting that by enterprise and improvisation he and Röntgen could become the leading men in their chosen field. If the Ministry of Education provided unlimited amounts of money for better laboratory equipment, Kundt went on, anyone, however lacking in ingenuity, could be a good physicist.

In 1872, Kundt was offered a post at the University at Strassburg, and once again he invited Röntgen to accompany him as his first assistant. The University, founded originally in 1567, had been virtually disbanded after the French Revolution, but it had been reopened after the Franco–Prussian War and the physicists were able to work, for a change, in a handsome and well-appointed building. Here, Röntgen found that as well as being a dedicated physicist he had a certain talent for teaching.

After three years at Strassburg, Röntgen was offered a full

professorship in physics and mathematics at the Agricultural Academy in Hohenheim, Württemberg. The appointment would mean breaking his close ties with Kundt, but Röntgen decided to accept the post. He found the facilities at Hohenheim wholly inadequate, however, and the apartments in which he lived with his young wife were overrun with rats and other vermin. So eighteen months later he readily accepted an invitation to return to Strassburg as an Assistant Professor of theoretical physics.

Throughout his years at Strassburg and at Hohenheim, Röntgen was concerned with the electromagnetic rotation of the plane of polarisation in gases. He enjoyed experimenting with crystals, too, because he believed that in these was to be found the embodiment of all natural laws. In all the papers he published on these and other subjects, Röntgen showed that under Kundt's scrupulous tuition he had become an ideal experimental physicist of the classical type. He saw clearly the nature of the problem he was studying; he carried out his experiments with great skill; and he conscientiously organised rigid control tests that would verify the results he had obtained. Finally, he would present his findings in a brief, precise and logical way.

By 1879, Röntgen's reputation had grown to such an extent that in that year he was recommended for the Chair of Physics at Geissen University. At Geissen, he was able to prove with the aid of a simply but extremely sensitive home-made thermometer that humid air can be heated more quickly than dry air, since water vapour actually absorbs heat radiation.

In 1880–1, Röntgen took over a new, well-equipped laboratory and lecture room. Here, he had the use of demonstration apparatus that he had designed and built himself. In the following years he developed his talent for measuring very small physical effects with meticulous accuracy, with the result that many of his findings have remained unchallenged to the present day.

By 1888, Röntgen had made for himself an international

reputation by proving that magnetic effects can be produced in a dielectric, such as a glass plate, if it is moved between two electrically charged condenser plates. Then, on 1 October of that year, he was offered the post of Professor of Physics and Director of the new physical institute of the University of Würzburg. Röntgen accepted eagerly. In the next six years he published no fewer than seventeen scientific papers.

The climax to Röntgen's scientific career came in the year 1895, when he found his attention virtually monopolised by the researches into cathode rays that were being carried out at that time by William Crookes (born 1832) in England, by Johann Wilhelm Hittorf (born 1824) in Germany, and by Philipp Eduard Anton Lenard (born 1862) who had been an assistant to the great physicist Heinrich Herz at the University of Bonn. With what was for him unusual single-mindedness, Röntgen decided to discontinue all his other researches and to devote himself exclusively to work of his own in this field.

He had obtained, already, from the glassblower Muller-Unkel of Braunschweig a tube of the type used by Lenard when the latter was observing the effects produced by passing powerful electric currents through free air and hydrogen. With this, some new Lenard tubes, a powerful induction coil that could produce sparks from four to six inches in length, and several Hittorf-Crookes tubes – 'discharge apparatus', Röntgen preferred to call these – Röntgen then equipped two laboratories on the first floor of his physical institute. He intended, with the apparatus, to study the results of passing high tension electric charges through highly evacuated vessels.

While he was repeating some of Lenard's earlier experiments, Röntgen enclosed an orthodox Lenard tube in a tightly fitting cardboard coat covered with tinfoil. Lenard had suggested that this should be done, to protect the thin aluminium window fitted to the tube from any damage that might possibly be caused by the powerful electrostatic field. At the same time, Lenard had said, the opaque jacket would prevent any light escaping visibly from the tube. With this covered tube, Röntgen was able to confirm, by his own observations, that invisible cathode rays did escape from the tube, as Lenard had suggested. More, they produced a fluorescent effect on a small cardboard screen that had been painted with barium platinocyanide, but they only did this if the screen were placed fairly close to the aluminium window of the tube. Fascinated by this, Röntgen decided to carry out some further experiments with a tube with heavier walls. With such a tube, he hazarded, it might be possible to produce fluorescent effects on the barium platinocyanide-coated screen even if the screen were placed at a much greater distance from the source of power.

Late on the afternoon of Friday 8 November 1895, when, as was his preference, he was working alone, Röntgen took a pear-shaped all-glass tube which had no thin metal window. He covered the tube with pieces of black cardboard, carefully cut and joined together to make a jacket similar to the one he had used previously on the Lenard tube. Next, he connected the tube with the electrodes of his powerful induction coil. After darkening the room so that he could test the opacity of the tube's black paper cover, Röntgen started the coil and passed a high tension discharge through the tube. He was pleased to see that no light, apparently, penetrated the cardboard cover.

Just as Röntgen was about to cut off the current so that he could set up the screen for the experiment he had planned, he noticed a strange, shimmering light that came from a top surface placed a little way from the apparatus with which he was working. To him, it looked as though some tiny ray of light had escaped from the tube or some small spark had escaped from the induction coil and was being reflected in a mirror or mirror-like surface.

At first, Röntgen was startled by this wholly unexpected phenomenon. Then, he passed another series of discharges through the tube. Each time, the same unexplained fluorescence appeared on the upper surface. In addition, Röntgen observed a faint cloud that appeared to move simultaneously with the fluctuating discharges of the coil.

In a state, by now, of considerable excitement, Röntgen struck a match. To his great surprise, he found that the mysterious glow was coming from the little screen, coated with barium platinocyanide, that he had left on a nearby table. So he repeated the experiment again and again, each time moving the screen a little further from the cathode ray tube. Each time, he obtained the same results.

Röntgen guessed that some other rays than cathode rays must be emanating from the Hittorf-Crookes tube, for Lenard had shown conclusively that cathode rays made free air electrically conductive, but he had also shown that they were totally absorbed after passing through only a few centimetres of that air. The new rays he had discovered were illuminating the barium platinocyanide-coated screen at distances of more than a metre.

Concentrating on his discovery, Röntgen became completely unaware of the passage of time and almost oblivious to his surroundings. The afternoon wore on; evening came; and several times his wife sent a servant to call him to dinner. When he finally sat down to his meal, he ate little and in almost complete silence. He made no reply when his wife asked him what the matter was. As quickly as possible, he returned to his laboratory. He spent the entire weekend there, repeating his experiments and systematically making notes on his observations.

In the weeks that followed, Röntgen worked feverishly in his laboratory. He had his meals taken in on a tray, and he had a small bed installed so that he could rest for a short time without leaving the place whenever he became completely exhausted. If the unknown rays he had discovered could penetrate a lightproof jacket and could penetrate air to a previously unobserved degree, he reasoned, there was a chance that they might also pass through other substances. To test the truth of his supposition, he held in turn a piece of paper, a playing card and a book between the tube and the illuminable screen. Each time he passed the current through the tube, the little screen would light up, though it did so rather less brightly when the rays were required to pass through the book. A thin sheet of aluminium decreased the degree of fluorescence on the screen about as effectively as had the book. A sheet of lead appeared to stop the fluorescence altogether.

While he was investigating the peculiar ability of lead to absorb, in some way, the unknown rays, Röntgen chose a small disc of lead and held it with his forefinger and thumb between the tube and the screen. To his amazement, he could see on the screen not only the round dark shadow of the lead but he could also distinguish the outlines of his thumb and finger. Inside these outlines, there were darker shadows – caused, it seemed almost certain, by the bones of his hand.

Throughout the last weeks of 1895, Röntgen worked in complete seclusion, trying to prove to his own satisfaction that his chance observation was, in fact, scientifically reliable. 'I have discovered something interesting', he told one of his trusted colleagues who had asked impatiently what was going on, 'but I do not know whether or not my observations are correct'.[1]

When he had proved that the newly-discovered emanations from the Hittorf-Crookes tube had the power to darken a photographic plate, Röntgen was able to extend his experiments. In one of these, he asked his wife to place her hand on a cassette loaded with a photographic plate, and on this he directed for fifteen minutes rays from his tube. When he had developed the plate, he saw the bones of his wife's hand depicted in light tones inside the darker shadows of the flesh that surrounded them. Two rings that she had on her fingers had almost completely stopped the rays, and were exactly silhouetted. When he showed his wife this plate, she was horrified by the thought that she was seeing her own skeleton.

Once he had proved to his own satisfaction that his observations were reliable, Röntgen lost no time in assembling

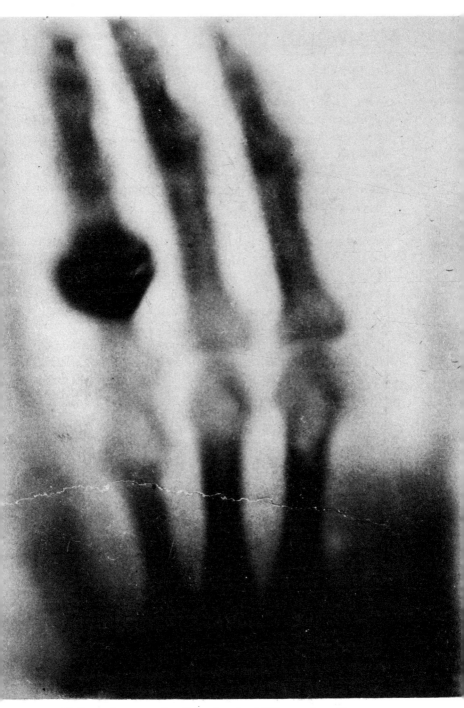

X-Ray photograph of the hand of Röntgen's wife

his notes. Shortly after Christmas 1895 he handed to the Secretary of the Würzburg Physical Medical Society the manuscript of a short paper called *On a New Kind of Rays, a Preliminary Communication*, asking that this should be published as quickly as possible in the transactions of the Society even though it had not been presented at a meeting of the Society in the usual way. Realising at once the extraordinary importance of Röntgen's paper, the Secretary arranged that it should be printed at once. By New Year's Day 1896, Röntgen was able to post copies of the paper to many reputable physicists, most of whom he regarded as his personal friends. He enclosed prints of the photographs of his wife's hand, and of other subjects that would demonstrate the scope and possible value of the newly-found rays. As he walked, carrying the packages, with his wife to the post box, he observed 'Now there will be the Devil to pay!'[2]

A flood of messages did, then, in fact, reach Röntgen from all over the world. Most of the writers congratulated him on a phenomenal discovery, though a few upbraided him for unleashing rays which would surely destroy all mankind.

On 9 January 1896, Röntgen received a telegraph from Kaiser Wilhelm II inviting him to demonstrate his world-stirring discovery at the Imperial Court. Protected from the severe winter weather by a heavy fur-lined coat and carrying a bulky brief case, Röntgen arrived at the royal castle late on the afternoon of 13 January 1896, apologising for his lack of punctuality with these words: 'I beg pardon, Your Majesty, for being late, but I am not used to these large distances here in Berlin'. After setting up his apparatus and demonstrating his new rays, Röntgen was decorated by the Emperor with the Prussian Order of the Crown, Second Class, and was invited to dine at the Imperial table.

When asked to lecture, on 23 January 1896, on his discovery by the members of the Würzburg Physical Medical Society, Röntgen asked Albert von Kölliker, the anatomist of the University, for permission to photograph his hand. Von Kölliker readily agreed. When, a little later, an excellent

X-ray picture of the anatomist's hand was shown to the audience, there was a storm of applause. The possibility of making such photographs of other parts of the human body was then eagerly discussed.[3]

The immense value of Röntgen's rays to all members of the medical profession was, after this, quickly seen, and surgeons in many different parts of the world were soon wanting shadow-pictures of broken bones and of serious dislocations. Bullets, shot, swallowed thimbles and other foreign bodies showed up well on the plates, it was found, and the rays could be used for finding and locating exactly stones in the kidney and other small natural annoyances that needed to be removed. Before long, the more advanced radiographers of the time were carrying out surveys of the human heart and lungs, which, being less dense than the relatively easily photographed bones around them, needed, for clarity, proportionately longer exposures.

No one could have welcomed Röntgen's discovery more heartily than did orthopaedic surgeons. Preoccupied as they were with fractures and other skeletal abnormalities, they had been seriously handicapped in their work, until then, by their inability to see under the skin. Robert Jones, nephew of the great Hugh Owen Thomas of Liverpool, was one of the first specialists in the world to appreciate the full significance of the Würzburg miracle.

In 1870, Hugh Owen Thomas offered to take his nephew, who was then thirteen years old, into his home. The uncle imposed a condition – the offer was made on the assumption that Robert would agree to study medicine. The boy accepted the offer, and three years later the youth arrived at the Thomas residence ready to enrol at the Liverpool School of Medicine. Five years after that, he graduated.

During the years of his apprenticeship, Robert Jones led a strange and exhausting existence, carrying out the arduous work of a medical student with the equally exacting tasks that fell to him as one of his distinguished uncle's principal assistants. Blessed with a formidably tough constitution,

Robert Jones managed to survive triumphantly this laborious training. In the process, he learned from his uncle how to combine a passion for public service with a complete disregard of his own personal needs.

When, in 1891, Hugh Owen Thomas died, quite worn out by his exceptional exertions, Robert Jones had to decide whether he ought to carry on with orthopaedic work or take an easier assignment in general surgery. Inevitably, Robert Jones chose the harder path – his loyalty to his uncle's memory left him no other comfortable option. He tried, as well as he could, to take his great predecessor's place.

Four years later, Robert Jones heard of the momentous discovery that William Conrad Röntgen had made at Würzburg. Having a lively and forward-looking mind, Robert Jones set off at once for Prussia to find out a bit more about Röntgen's researches. Having heard Röntgen's story and having seen a demonstration of his extraordinary flesh-penetrating process, the young Welshman ordered and paid for an X-ray tube. Then he returned to England, and there he and another young man called Thurston Holland, later to become one of Britain's most eminent radiologists, took an X-ray photograph. It was almost certainly the first X-ray picture to be taken anywhere in the British Isles. The photograph showed plainly a small bullet that was embedded deeply in a boy's wrist. Looking at it, Robert Jones realised at once how immensely valuable X-ray photography would be to all future orthopaedic surgeons, and to so many other medical men and women besides. But he did not allow his judgement to become clouded by the excitements roused by Röntgen's new technique. Jones knew only too well how dangerous were all modern short cuts to genuine scientific knowledge. 'While Röntgen's discovery has been to us of immense value, chiefly in the classification of our injuries', he wrote, 'it has done little if anything to perfect or alter our treatment of fractures'. All medical students should acquire proper clinical skills in diagnosis, he went on. They should not rely exclusively on the interpretation of a fallible photograph.

Robert Jones's verdict on the new X-rays is still upheld today. His reservations did not lessen the respect with which Röntgen was internationally regarded, though. In 1901, Röntgen was awarded the first Nobel Prize for physics.

# 16

# The Discovery of Radium

. . . 'It was a maxim of Captain Swosser's', said Mrs
Badger, 'speaking in his figurative naval manner, that
when you make pitch hot, you cannot make it too hot;
and that if you only have to swab a plank, you should
swab it as if Davy Jones were after you . . .'

CHARLES DICKENS, Bleak House

Marie Curie, one of the world's most dedicated scientists, was
born in Warsaw on 7 November 1867. Her name, during the
early years of her life, was Manya Sklodowska.

While she was still a child, Manya attracted the attention of
many adults by her unusual intellectual powers and by her
prodigious memory. She could read easily by the time she
was four, and that was before her elder sister Bronia had
learned to put two or three cardboard letters together to
make a simple one-syllable word. But Manya Sklodowska
was being brought up in an occupied country. Russian
inspectors would enter her school unexpectedly, hoping to
catch the pupils studying Polish history and literature instead
of the Russian history and literature that the authorities
required. Long before she became a senior student, Manya
had learned how to put her work quietly away when any
unannounced visitor appeared on the school premises.

By the time she was sixteen, Manya had been awarded a
gold medal for her academic achievements. She had learned,
too, how to get her own way in spite of all prevailing
difficulties. Many of the difficulties Manya had to face were
the result of her unfortunate family circumstances. Her
mother had died and her father, a teacher of mathematics and
physics, had lost most of his money through unwise

investment. He was not earning a large salary and when he was due to retire could only expect a very small pension. So Manya was compelled to give lessons, for small payments, to children of the better-off. There were few other opportunities in Poland in those days for women to earn money honestly. While she was not actually teaching, the girl worked conscientiously for an 'underground' university, the patriotic members of which would read, in Polish, to less well-educated workers in an attempt to make them resist more effectively the pressures that were being applied to them by their Russian overlords.

Manya might have continued as a freelance teacher in Poland for the rest of her life, or at least until she married, but her horizons were widened considerably when her sister Bronia decided to travel to Paris to study medicine. Unselfishly, Manya offered to give Bronia her small savings and all the money she would earn in the near future as a governess on the understanding that Bronia would, later, help her in much the same way. A succession of more lucrative engagements followed for Manya. Hired by the members of very wealthy families, she was able to experience for the first time the advantages of living in comfortable homes, where the presence of beautiful furniture and pictures was taken for granted. In no way overawed by all this unaccustomed luxury, Manya was much more impressed by the little Museum of Industry and Agriculture in Warsaw, which the Russians, believing it to be only of limited interest to the Poles, had not closed. Of this museum, one of Manya's cousins happened to be the Director. Secretly, in the museum, this cousin was giving science lessons. For the first time in her life, Manya was able to enter a laboratory and to handle scientific instruments. Before long, she was trying, unaided, to reproduce the experiments she had seen described in her school textbooks. She was fascinated. Her ambition – to get to Paris as quickly as she could, and to study there – became really urgent. Soon she was writing to her sister in Paris asking that she should be accommodated there, and promising to be no trouble whatsoever.

So in 1891 the young Polish woman set off for Paris, her bedding and a few other simple necessities having been sent on in advance by freight train. She travelled in the cheapest possible way in 'fourth class' trucks that had no seats other than hard benches attached to the four sides. When she arrived in Paris she started to attend lectures at the Sorbonne, finding at first that her limited knowledge of the French language was a severe handicap. In spite of this, her unusual abilities were quickly recognised and she was soon asked to carry out a programme of original research. Then, in order that she might be able to concentrate on her work with fewer distractions than she could expect at the comfortable sub- urban home of her sister and brother-in-law, she took a room of her own. And she started to call herself 'Marie', the French name by which, with the new surname she acquired when she was married, she is universally remembered today.

The conditions under which Marie Sklodowska managed to exist in her bare garret room in the students' quarter of Paris were austere. She had no gas to provide heat or light. Her only water supply came from a tap on the landing which she shared with the other tenants of the house. As soon as daylight started to fade, she would go to the nearby library of Ste Geneviève, and there she would continue her studies until the library closed, two hours before midnight. She would then return to her attic each night for another four hours' work carried out by the light of a single small oil lamp. Two hours after midnight she would cease studying and would go, mentally exhausted, to bed. She was much too preoccupied with her work to bother about food. Usually she managed to keep herself alive with slices of bread and butter, varied occasionally with some luxurious addition such as a boiled egg or a saucerful of cherries. More than once, her brother- in-law found Marie in a state of collapse and then she would have to be taken back to the comfort of her sister's home so that she could be nursed back to health. It was a way of life that could well have killed a less formidable person. Marie

Sklodowska appeared to thrive just sufficiently on it to be able to graduate in physics in 1893. She came first of all the students in this subject at the Sorbonne, and she graduated in mathematics in 1894, though in this subject she managed only to achieve second place.

In 1894, she met Pierre Curie, and an important new phase in her life began.

Pierre Curie had been born in Paris on 15 May 1859. His father was a physician, and Pierre had soon shown his parents that he was a very unusual child. When he was only fourteen, he spent most of his spare time working out problems in spatial geometry. He had matriculated at the Sorbonne when he was sixteen, and before he was twenty he had obtained his Licence ès Sciences which is roughly equivalent to the Bachelor of Science degree. In the same year, 1878, he had started his first really important piece of research which concerned the calculation of the wavelength of heat waves. By the time Marie Sklodowska was introduced to him by mutual friends, Curie had been appointed Supervisor of the School of Physics and Industrial Chemistry in Paris. She had been asked by the officials of the Society for the Encouragement of National Industry to prepare a thesis on the magnetic properties of different kinds of steel and she needed more working space than she could be given in the laboratories of her own professor. Would M. Curie let her bring the heavy apparatus she needed into his school, she asked? The answer was 'Yes', and before many months had elapsed the two scientists had become engaged.

The marriage of Pierre Curie and Marie Sklodowska on 25 July 1895 marked the official start of a working partnership that was soon to be of international importance. From the beginning, Marie managed to keep house economically and to continue her scientific researches with equal success. Then came a baby daughter – Irene – and the child added considerably to Marie's domestic responsibilities. Undeterred, she decided to work hard to obtain a doctorate, a distinction coveted by virtually every scientist of the time. To succeed, she knew that she would have to make some major contribution to scientific knowledge. In what field, she wondered, should her researches be carried out?

While talking the matter over with her husband, Marie Curie was reminded of something that he, and she, had read a little time before. In a journal in which the latest scientific discoveries were regularly discussed, a man named Henri Becquerel had described a phenomenon that appeared to be quite new. While studying the rare metal uranium, Becquerel had written, he had found that the salts of the metal gave off, spontaneously, rays similar to the X-rays that William Conrad Röntgen had discovered only a short time before. More, he had found that electrically charged bodies were discharged if they were exposed to gases through which those rays were passing. Marie Curie, intrigued by the extraordinary radiation that Becquerel had discovered, decided to find out as much as she could about it. If she managed to find out the cause of the radiation and its nature, she realised, she could make her researches the subject of the doctor's thesis she so badly wanted to write. Her husband agreed, and Marie prepared to start work.

First, she knew, she would need floor space, and plenty of it. But there was no suitable workshop to be found. Then the Director of the School of Physics suggested that she might like to use for her researches an old store room on the ground floor of his premises. It was cold and dirty and damp and partly filled with disused equipment, but Marie Curie took it and there she set up her electroscope and other necessary appliances. By looking with a microscope through a hole in the case of her electroscope, after the electroscope had been charged, Marie Curie could watch the behaviour of a strip of gold leaf. By the movements of the gold leaf, she could judge how quickly the charge of the electroscope was leaking away. By using, in conjunction with this piece of apparatus, specimens of material containing uranium, she was able to establish beyond doubt, before many weeks had elapsed, that the ray-giving quality of the specimens she had selected was in direct proportion to the quantity of pure uranium they contained. But she could find out little else about the essential nature of this strange radiance by studying only uranium. Was there any possibility, she wondered, that radiance of the same kind could be found in any other substance?

With characteristic dedication, Marie Curie then set herself the task of testing for the radiance, in her revealing electroscope, every known chemical substance. She was determined to do this without neglecting her husband, her baby, or her increasing domestic responsibilities. Before long, she had found that a substance named thorium was also 'radioactive', as she decided to call the rare quality in which she had become so interested. A German scientist named Gerhard Carl Schmidt discovered the unusual nature of thorium at approximately the same time.

Knowing for certain that two positively-identified chemical substances, and as far as she could see only two, were radioactive, Marie Curie then tried to find some explanation of their apparently unique power. Examining methodically, in her attempt to find out more about the spontaneous light-giving capacities of uranium and thorium, every mineral known to contain the slightest trace of either of them, she then discovered to her surprise that the minerals chalcolite and pitchblende (a native oxide of uranium, found usually in blackish pitch-like masses) appeared to be more radioactive than uranium itself. When she announced her findings, on 12 April 1898, she declared her belief that these minerals might contain an element, previously unknown, which would prove to be more radioactive than uranium.

Marie Curie's momentous announcement helped to divert her husband's interest from his own researches, and from then on the two worked together on the historic task of isolating, if they could, Marie's 'new element'. They would need for their experiments, they saw, large quantities of pitchblende. They might have felt discouraged if they had known, at that stage in their work, that the mysterious substance for which they were looking would represent only about one-millionth part of every load of pitchblende they would have to order.

By July 1898, Pierre and Marie Curie had decided that there were two radioactive ingredients of pitchblende, not one. The first they could identify, and Marie gave it the name polonium, as a respectful tribute to her native country. The second was much more difficult to isolate, but by December in the same year they felt confident enough to be able to write of it, in a paper they prepared for the Academy of Science: 'The new radioactive substance contains a new element to which we propose to give the name radium. The radio-activity of radium must be enormous'.

To establish the existence of radium with sufficient certainty to convince even the most sceptical of scientists, the Curies saw that they would have to extract, somehow, from pitchblende a sample that would be large enough to be weighed, since no reputable scientist would be prepared to believe in the existence of any material, however well vouched for by other experts it might be, unless its atomic weight were known.

Where, they wondered, could they get enough pitchblende for what they needed to do? To extract from a mass of pitchblende sufficient radium to be seen and weighed, that mass of pitchblende might have to weigh several tons. Where could they possibly obtain several tons of it? How could they possibly pay for it, if they could find it, or store it, if they could find it and if they could pay for it? How, if they could find, pay for, and store so much pitchblende, could they work on it so that it would yield the radium that Marie Curie believed it contained?

They soon found the answer to the first of those questions. In Bohemia, now part of Czechoslovakia, glass-manufactur-ers bought huge quantities of pitchblende, extracted from it the uranium they needed for their glass-factories, and then threw the residue away in the Forest of St Joachimstal, so that the forest was disfigured by heaps of powdery brown waste. The glass-manufacturers did not expect to receive any finan-

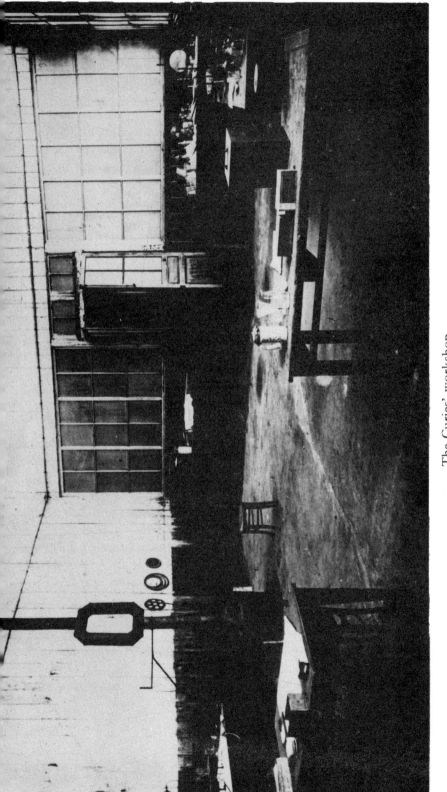

The Curies' workshop

cial reward for the material they had thrown away – but they did ask Pierre and Marie Curie to pay the cost of transporting the apparently valueless dust to France. The Curies did not at that time have much spare money, but they dug as deeply as they dared into their small savings and asked that several railway wagons should be filled with the stuff and that the wagons should then be dispatched, as quickly as possible, to Paris. They had nowhere suitable to put the dust, once it arrived – there were no spare rooms in the Sorbonne, or in the School of Physics. Instead, the Curies had to arrange for the mixture of unwanted powder and Bohemian pine needles to be delivered to an entirely unsuitable shed near Pierre Curie's school – a shed with a glass roof that leaked badly whenever rain fell on it, and with an uneven floor; a shed that would be tormentingly hot in the summer months and almost unbearably cold in the depths of winter; a shed fitted with no devices whatsoever for the disposal of poisonous fumes; a shed, in short, that no reasonable scientist would have looked at for a moment if there had been any clean, temperate and weatherproof alternative within reach. The Curies, having no alternative, had to settle for that unsatisfactory shed.

The pitchblende arrived at the shed in large sacks that were carried on horse-drawn vehicles normally used for the delivery of coal. Marie Curie, waiting eagerly to receive the precious dust, opened one of the sacks in the street before it had been taken off the wagon. She plunged her fingers into the apparently inert dun-coloured powder. In it, she felt sure, was the mysterious substance that posed one of the great unanswered questions of the universe. It was up to her to isolate that substance and force it to give her a proper explanation of its power.

During the next few years Marie Curie laboured, without allowing herself any adequate rest, on her gigantic task. There was, she felt sure, some substance in the pitchblende that could be concentrated with barium and then separated from the surrounding material by a laborious process of **fractional crystallisation**.

First, she had a bulky iron cauldron set up in the yard by her radium shed and by it, enveloped in acrid smoke, she would spend most of her days stirring, with an iron poker that was almost as long as she was, the unattractive brown fluids that her 'saucepan' contained. Clad in a dirty overall that would often be spattered with acids, she would sometimes be dealing with as much as forty pounds of the pitchblende. She would lift heavy pots, without aid, as cheerfully as would any muscular workman. However tired she became, she refused to give up or to work more slowly. Before long, the old tables in the workshed were loaded with vessels that contained samples of increasingly concentrated products – substances which, as the months passed, were richer and richer in radium. Pierre Curie, working with almost as much determination as his wife, was carrying out meanwhile many delicate and protracted experiments that were intended to establish, scientifically, the true properties of radium. Time and time again, further supplies of pitchblende had to be sent for from Bohemia.

For more than three years, Marie Curie worked away at the purification and fractional crystallisation of her solutions, but eventually the difficulties under which she was labouring began to seem insurmountable. Urgently needing a spotlessly clean and well-insulated working place for the remaining processes of her great work, she was forced to continue in the draughty, dirty shed in which she had begun, and the repeated intrusion of unwanted iron and coal dust and other impurities into her precious fluids drove her almost to despair. Seeing his wife compelled to repeat so much of her work because it had been spoiled in this way, Pierre Curie did urge her, in fact, to give up her attempts to prepare pure radium until she could resume her struggles under less daunting conditions, but Marie Curie was obdurate. She was determined to finish as quickly as possible what she had set out to do.

More obstacles followed. With a growing child to care for, the Curies needed more money than their scientific researches

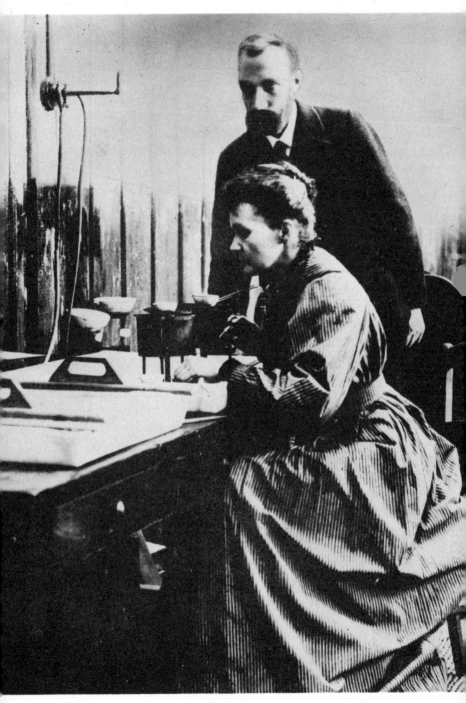

The Curies at work

could at that time possibly earn them, and they were forced to waste many precious hours on activities that had nothing to do with the isolation of radium. Pierre Curie had to take on a humble but demanding post as a tutor at the Paris 'Polytechnique'; Marie started to teach girls in a training school for elementary teachers at Sèvres, which was a long tram-ride away from her little home at 108 Boulevard Killermann and a million miles away, in spirit, from her normal working place. Insufficiently fed and, in consequence, in ever-present danger of becoming seriously ill, Marie Curie continued to work, in every possible waking moment, on her radium researches.

At long last, in 1902, forty-five months after the day on which Pierre and Marie Curie had announced the probable existence of radium, Marie succeeded triumphantly in the task to which she had devoted so many hours and so much energy. She managed, against all the odds, to prepare one decigramme of pure radium. More, she was able to determine radium's atomic weight. (This is given in her daughter's account of the great discovery as '225'.) Also included in Eve Curie's classic biography of her mother is a striking description of the visit that Pierre and Marie Curie made to their workshop just after Marie had achieved the apparently impossible:

> Old Dr. Curie [Pierre Curie's father], who lived with the couple, had retired to his room. Marie had bathed her child and put her to bed, and had stayed for a long time beside the cot. This was a rite. When Irene did not feel her mother near her at night she would call out for her incessantly, with that 'Mé!' which was to be our substitute for 'Mamma' always. And Marie, yielding to the implacability of the four-year-old child, climbed the stairs, seated herself beside her and stayed there in the darkness until the young voice gave way to light, regular breathing. Only then would she go down again to Pierre, who was growing impatient.
>
> The day's work had been hard, and it would have been

more reasonable for the couple to rest. As soon as they had put on their coats and told Dr. Curie of their flight, they were in the street. They were on foot, arm in arm, exchanging few words. After the crowded streets of this queer district, with its factory buildings, waste-lands and poor tenements, they arrived in the Rue Lhomond and crossed the little courtyard. Pierre put the key in the lock. The door squeaked, as it had squeaked thousands of times, and admitted them to their realm, to their dream.

'Don't light the lamps!' Marie said in the darkness. Then she added with a little laugh: 'Do you remember the day when you said to me "I should like radium to have a beautiful colour"?'

The reality was more entrancing than the simple wish of long ago. Radium had something better than 'a beautiful colour'; it was spontaneously luminous. And in the sombre shed, where, in the absence of cupboards, the precious particles in their tiny glass receivers were placed on tables or on shelves nailed to the wall, their phosphorescent bluish outlines gleamed, suspended in the night.

'Look . . . Look!' the young woman murmured.

She went forward cautiously, looked for and found a straw-bottomed chair. She sat down in the darkness and silence. Their two faces turned towards the pale glimmering, the mysterious sources of radiation, toward radium – their radium. Her body leaning forward, her head eager, Marie took up again the attitude which had been hers an hour earlier at the bedside of her sleeping child.

Her companion's hand lightly touched her hair.

She was to remember for ever this evening of glow-worms, this magic . . .

News of the Curies' achievement spread rapidly after that to all parts of the world. Scientists everywhere appreciated some, if not all, of the significance of the French couple's discovery and many planned at once to start working with radium and with the substances that were most nearly related to it. The British scientist Sir William Ramsay, assisted by Frederick Soddy, was quick to discover that radium gave off from itself minute quantities of a previously unknown gas which they called helium. And other people beside scientists were made aware of the Curies and their historic researches. The fact that a woman was capable of such a feat was enough, at that time, to cause an international sensation.

Sensations of a different kind were caused when Pierre Curie, still carrying on his researches, noticed that the skin of one of his hands was becoming red, as if it had been burned. Twenty days later, a scab appeared on the affected place, and this was followed by some soreness. On the forty-second day after the start of the trouble, the sore began to heal at its outside edge. Marie, too, found radium 'burns' on herself, though the substance that appeared to have done the damage to her was safely – as she thought – enclosed in a glass tube which, in its turn, was shut away in a tin box. Most alarming of all the injuries experienced in the very early days of radium were those suffered by the Curies' friend and colleague Henri Becquerel. When Becquerel carried in his pocket a tube containing radium he found that he was quite seriously affected.

Soon, the burns suffered by the Curies and by Becquerel were attracting the attention of forward-looking members of the medical profession. Why, these doctors wondered, did radium burns heal so well? Might not radium be useful for burning away diseased skin and other unwanted tissues? Might not radium be useful for treating cancer which was, and still is, one of mankind's most puzzling diseases?

When Marie Curie was awarded, in 1903, half the Nobel Prize for Science – Henri Becquerel was awarded the other half – those ready to carry out research into the medical potentialities of radium were given the most effective encouragement. The founding of the Radium Hospital in Paris in 1906 opened a new chapter in the history of the treatment of human malignancies.

# Notes and Sources

*Chapter 1*

Principal sources: Fielding H. Garrison, A.B., M.D., *An Introduction to the History of Medicine*, W.B. Saunders Company, Philadelphia and London, 1913; Douglas Guthrie, M.D., F.R.C.S. [Ed.], F.R.S.E., *A History of Medicine*, Thomas Nelson and Sons Ltd, London, 1945; and Wyndham E.B. Lloyd, *A Hundred Years of Medicine (Second Edition)*, Duckworth and Company, London, 1968.

1  The three Alexander Monros were responsible for the teaching of anatomy at Edinburgh University over a continuous period of 126 years.

*Chapter 2*

Principal sources: S. Foart Simmons, *Account of the Life and Writings of William Hunter*, 1783; Sir E. Home, *Life of Dr John Hunter prefixed to Hunter's Treatise on the Blood, etc.*, 1794; Drewry Ottley, *Life of Dr John Hunter*, 1835; and Dr John Thomson, *An Account of the Life, Lectures and Writings of William Cullen*, Edinburgh, 1832.

1  William Cullen's clinical lectures were delivered in English: not, like most other medical lectures of the day, in Latin.

2  On 5 July 1755, at the University of Oxford, John Hunter was matriculated as a Commoner of St Mary Hall. His name was kept on the books there until December 1756, but the dour young Scotsman does not seem to have approved of higher education of the Oxford kind, for in later life he told Sir

Anthony Carlisle 'They wanted to make an old woman of me, or that I should stuff Latin and Greek at the University, but', he added emphatically, pressing his thumb nail on the table, 'these schemes I cracked like so many vermin as they came before me'.

*Chapter 3*

Principal sources: Simmons's *Life of William Hunter*, London, 1783; Pettigrew's *Memoirs of John Coakley Lettsom*, London, 1817; John Baron, *Life of Edward Jenner*, 1838; B.B. Cooper, *Life of Sir Astley Paston Cooper*, London, 1843; Macilwain's *Memoirs of John Abernethy*, London, 1853; G.T. Bettany's *Eminent Doctors*, 1885.

1  S.D. Gross [Ed.], *Lives of Eminent American Physicians and Surgeons*, Philadelphia, 1861.
2  G. Edwards, *Philip Syng Physick, 1768–1837*, Proceedings of the Royal Society of Medicine, 1940.
3  In *The Age of Agony*, Constable and Company, London, 1975.
4  Bettany.
5  J.C. Jeaffreson, *A Book about Doctors*, 1870.
6  When he died, on 12 February 1841, in his seventy-third year, Sir Astley Cooper was buried, at his express wish, in the chapel at Guy's Hospital.
7  J. Forbes, *On Percussion of the Chest: A Translation of Auenbrugger's Original Treatise*, Bulletin of Historical Medicine, 1936.
8  H. Saintignon, *Laënnec, Sa Vie et Son Oeuvre*, Paris, 1904.
9  Sir W. Hale-White, *Laënnec: Translation of Selected Passages from 'De L'Auscultation Médiate' with a Biography*, 1923.

*Chapter 4*

Principal sources: *The Trial of William Burke*, 1829, Famous British Trials Series; *The Newgate Calendar*; Sir John Bowring, *Jeremy Bentham's Life and Works*, 1843.

1  *The Trial of William Burke*.
2  Ibid.

*Chapter 5*

Principal sources: John Davy, *Memoirs of the Life of Sir Humphry Davy, Bart.*; John Davy [Ed.], *Fragmentary Remains, Literary and Scientific, of Sir Humphry Davy*; Weld's *History of the Royal Society*; *The Times*, 20 December 1847; John Snow, *Chloroform and Other Anaesthetics*, edited, with a Memoir, by B.W. Richardson, London, 1858; John Duns, D.D., *A Memoir of Sir James Young Simpson*, Edinburgh, 1873; H.B. McCall, *Some Old Families: A Contribution to the Genealogical History of Scotland*, 1890; *Joseph Toynbee, a Memoir* by G.T. Bettany in *Eminent Doctors*.

1   Davy, *Memoirs*.
2   Ibid.
3   Ibid.
4   Ibid.
5   Ibid.
6   Ibid.
7   Ibid.
8   Ibid.
9   Ibid.
10  Ibid.
11  Dictionary of National Biography.
12  Garrison, *Introduction to the History of Medicine*.
13  Wells's personality seems to have been radically changed by his inhalation of chemical vapours, for he was eventually jailed, in New York, for throwing acid at passers-by. He took his own life in a prison cell while the members of the Paris Medical Society were publicly acclaiming him as the discoverer of anaesthetic gases.
14  Garrison.
15  Garrison.
16  Duns, *A Memoir*.
17  Ibid.

*Chapter 6*

Principal sources: Lord Lister, *Collected Papers*, Oxford, 1909;

R. J. Godlee, *Lord Lister*, Oxford, 1924; W. Cheyne, *Lister and his Achievement*, 1925; A. Turner, *Joseph, Baron Lister, Centenary Volume*, Edinburgh, 1927.

1  Godlee, *Lord Lister*.
2  J.D. Comrie, *History of Scottish Medicine*, 1932.
3  *Collected Papers*, Oxford, 1909.
4  Godlee, *Lord Lister*.
5  Ibid.
6  Royal Commission, *Minutes of Evidence*, London, 1876.
7  Douglas Guthrie, M.D., F.R.C.S., in his *A History of Medicine* (Thomas Nelson and Sons, London, 1945) seems to suggest that Joseph Lister and his wife carried flasks of 'urine' around in cabs and railway carriages. If the lecture notes taken by William Stirling Anderson, one of Lister's students, are studied carefully, it may be seen that the liquid was, in fact, wine.
8  Godlee, *Lord Lister*.
9  Ibid.
10  Ibid.

*Chapter 7*

Principal sources: Schuerer Von Waldheim, *Ignaz Philipp Semmelweis*, 1905; George Frederic Still, M.A., M.D., Hon. LL.D., F.R.C.P., *The History of Paediatrics*, Oxford University Press, 1931; Erwin H. Ackernecht, *A Short History of Medicine*, Ronald Press Co., New York, 1955.

1  A number of maternity hospitals had existed in London since the eighteenth century, but they were primarily intended for married women. (The City of London Lying-In Hospital, founded in 1750, was one of these.) If such hospitals accepted unmarried mothers, the patients were invariably subjected to rigorous conditions. The New Westminster Lying-In Hospital (founded in 1767) accepted 'women such as are deserted and in deep distress, to save them from despair and the lamentable crimes of suicide and child murder'. The Clapham Maternity Hospital (founded in 1889) accepted only 'the better class of unmarried girls'.

*Chapter 8*

Principal sources: Lord Stanmore, *Lord Herbert of Lea*, 1906;
M.A. Nutting and L.L. Dock, *History of Nursing*, New York,
1907; *The Times*, 14–23 August 1910; Cecil Woodham-Smith,
*Florence Nightingale*, Constable and Company, London, 1950.

1 Woodham-Smith, *Florence Nightingale*.
2 Ibid.
3 Ibid.
4 Ibid.
5 Ibid.
6 Ibid.
7 Ibid.
8 Ibid.
9 Ibid.
10 Ibid.
11 Ibid.
12 *The Times*.
13 Woodham-Smith, *Florence Nightingale*.
14 Ibid.
15 Ibid.
16 Ibid.
17 Ibid.
18 Ibid.
19 Ibid.
20 Ibid.
21 Ibid.
22 Ibid.
23 Ibid.
24 Ibid.
25 Ibid.
26 Ibid.
27 *Country Life*, 4 November 1976.
28 Woodham-Smith, *Florence Nightingale*.
29 Ibid.
30 Ibid.

*Chapter 9*

Principal sources: Frederick Watson, *Hugh Owen Thomas*,

Oxford University Press, 1934; David Le Vay, *The Life of Hugh Owen Thomas*, E. & S. Livingstone Ltd, Edinburgh and London, 1956.

1    Consular papers.
2    Watson, *Hugh Owen Thomas*.
3    Ibid.
4    F. Watson, *The Life of Sir Robert Jones*, London, 1934.
5    Watson, *Hugh Owen Thomas*.
6    Sir Robert Jones, *Memoirs*.


*Chapter 10*

Principal sources: An obituary notice of Doctor Alexander Wood in *The Edinburgh Medical Journal*, 1883–4; *Journal of The Johns Hopkins Hospital, Baltimore*; Geoffrey Keynes [Ed.] *Blood Transfusion*, John Wright and Sons, Bristol, and Simpkin Marshall Ltd, London, 1949.

1    Referred to by William Shakespeare in *Julius Caesar*:
                                        . . .Stoop, Romans, stoop,
     And let us bathe our hands in Caesar's blood
     Up to the elbows . . .
2    Keynes [Ed.], *Blood Transfusion*.


*Chapter 11*

Principal sources: A.B. Granville, *The Spas of England*, 1841; *Medical Reflections on the Water Cure*, 1842; William MacLeod, *Directory of Ben Rhydding*, 1852; John Smedley, *Practical Hydropathy*, 1858; Henry Steer, *The Smedleys of Matlock Bank*, 1897; E.S. Turner, *Taking the Cure*, Michael Joseph, London, 1967.

1    Turner, *Taking the Cure*.
2    The long title of this work continued: 'with Advice to the Water Drinkers at Tunbridge Wells, Hampstead, Astrope, Nasborough and All the Other Chalybeate Spaws Wherein the Usefulness of Cold Bathing is Further Recommended to the Lovers of Coffee, Tea, Chocolate, Brandy, Etc.'
3    'Cold bathing has this good alone,

It makes Old John to hug Old Joan,
And gives a sort of resurrection
To buried joys, through lost erection,
And does fresh kindnesses entail,
On a wife tasteless, old and stale'.
Eighteenth-century jingle.

4   Frederic C. Coley, *The Turkish Bath*, 1887.
5   Ibid.


*Chapter 12*

Principal sources: P.H. Manson-Bahr and A. Alcock, *The Life and Work of Sir Patrick Manson*, 1927; Sir Ronald Ross, *Memoirs*, 1923; The League of Nations Health Organisation, *Further Report on Tuberculosis and Sleeping Sickness*, Geneva, 1925; R.L. Megroz, *Sir Ronald Ross: Discoverer and Creator*, 1931.

1   Manson died in London on 9 April 1922 and was buried in the Allenvale Cemetery in Aberdeen.


*Chapter 13*

Principal sources: John S. Rowntree, *Memoir of Samuel Tuke, Friends' Quarterly Examiner*, April 1895; D. Hack Tuke, *History of the Insane in the British Islands*, 1882; J.M. Charcot, *Clinical Lectures on the Diseases of the Nervous System*, New Sydenham Society, London, 1889; J.M. Charcot and Pierre Marie [Edited by D. Hack Tuke], *Hysteria* in *The Dictionary of Psychological Medicine*, Churchill, London, 1892; C. Lloyd Tuckey, *Treatment by Hypnotism and Suggestion*, Bailliere, Tyndall and Cox, London, 1900; Sigmund Freud, *Charcot: Collected Papers*, Hogarth Press, London, 1948; Georges Guillain, *J.M. Charcot, His Life, His Work*, Pitman Medical Publishing Company, London, 1959; A.R.G. Owen, *Hysteria, Hypnosis and Healing: The Work of J.M. Charcot*, Dennis Dobson, London, 1971.

1   The caring of friends gives proof of humanity.
2   John S. Rowntree, *Memoir of S. Tuke.*
3   Ibid.
4   Münthe.

5  J.M. Charcot, *Clinical Lectures.*
6  Ibid.
7  Ibid.
8  S. Freud, *Charcot: Collected Papers.*
9  J.M. Charcot, *Clinical Lectures.*
10  Ibid.
11  *J.M. Charcot, His Life.*
12  S. Freud, *Charcot, Collected Papers.*


*Chapter 14*

Principal sources: *Annual Register*, 1883; *Illustrated London News*, 5 January 1884; *The Times*, 8 April 1907; *Chemist and Druggist*, 13 April 1907; Stanley Chapman, *Jesse Boot of Boots the Chemists*, Hodder and Stoughton, London, 1974; G. Ruthven Mitchell, *Homoeopathy*, W. H. Allen, London, 1975.

1  A small plant, *Cuminum Cyminum*, bearing aromatic, seed-like fruit used in cookery and medicine.
2  They excused from their ban country doctors living too far from any town to get their prescriptions properly and legally made up.
3  Stanley Chapman, *Jesse Boot of Boots the Chemists.*


*Chapter 15*

Principal sources: F. Watson, *The Life of Sir Robert Jones*, London, 1934; Otto Glasser, Ph.D., F.A.C.R. (Assoc.), *Dr. W.C. Röntgen*, Charles C. Thomas, Springfield, Illinois, 1945; W. Robert Nitske, *The Life of William Conrad Röntgen, Discoverer of the X Ray*, University of Arizona Press, 1971.

1  W.R. Nitske, *The Life of William Conrad Röntgen.*
2  Ibid.
3  It was decided at this meeting that the new rays should be called 'Röntgen rays'. Their discoverer, realising that he was still unaware of the true nature of the rays, preferred that they should be called 'X-rays' – the name normally given to them today.

*Chapter 16*

Principal source: Ève Curie, *Madame Curie*, English translation, Heinemann, London, 1939.

# *Index*